Y0-BDA-755

General Systems Theory Applied to Nursing

General Systems Theory Applied to Nursing

Arlene M. Putt, R.N., Ed.D.
Professor of Nursing,
The University of Arizona College of Nursing, Tucson

Little, Brown and Company Boston

First Edition

Library of Congress Catalog Card No. 78-50620

ISBN 0-316-72300-2

Printed in the United States of America

To my mother, Mary E. Putt,
for her constant support over the years

Preface

The ideas presented here are derived from nine years of teaching in graduate education in nursing. June C. Abbey, Ph.D., now Professor of Nursing at the University of Utah, first introduced me to the concepts of general systems theory. General systems theory was developed by Ludwig von Bertalanffy, who attempted to formulate principles common to diverse systems encountered in a wide variety of scientific disciplines. From the ideas adopted by Dr. Abbey, I applied the concepts of general systems theory to the developing master's program in medical-surgical nursing at the University of Arizona College of Nursing, Tucson. The rewards were great.

To date, nine groups of students in this master's program have encountered general systems theory in the nursing context. Some of the students tried the concepts and then passed on to other frames of reference. The majority found the application of this theory very well suited to the assessment of nursing needs, the development of nursing care plans, and the determination of nursing actions. Exposure to general systems theory enriched the students' thought processes, and many students stated that their skill in solving problems had been enhanced through this experience. Because general systems theory thus proved valuable for nursing education, I was encouraged to explain and expand its application so that others might share this wealth of thought.

This theoretical framework can also be a very useful tool for the nursing practitioner who is in the process of expanding her role and responsibilities. It utilizes a taxonomy of the nursing process from assessment to evaluation, a cycle that is reviewed and repeated as needed. The nursing care plans growing out of general systems theory also form a guideline for adequate recording of care and could be a useful tool in nursing audits. The ideas and uses for general systems theory continue to multiply. You, the reader, must decide how useful the ideas presented here are to your own conceptual framework for nursing. The true test of a theory is whether it can withstand the rigors of application over time. Therefore, usage will be the measure of how valuable general systems theory will be to nursing.

A. M. P.

Contributing Authors

June C. Abbey, R.N., Ph.D., F.A.A.N.
Director, Physiological Nursing Program,
College of Nursing, The University of Utah,
Salt Lake City, Utah

Linda L. Brommer Bustamante, R.N., M.S.N.
Nursing Unit Director, Medical Service,
St. Mary's Hospital,
Tucson, Arizona

Mary Ellen Hazzard, R.N., M.Ed., M.S.
Assistant Professor of Psychiatric Nursing,
College of Nursing, The University of Arizona,
Tucson, Arizona

Ellen Kval Isaak, R.N., M.S.
Lecturer,
College of Nursing, The University of Arizona,
Tucson, Arizona

Peggy Sue MacMacken, M.S.N.
Clinical Nurse Specialist, Nursing Service,
St. Joseph's Hospital,
Tucson, Arizona

Deborah L. Oakes, R.N., M.S.N.
Staff Nurse, Surgical Intensive Care Unit,
Veterans Administration Hospital,
Tampa, Florida

Roberta Ann Palmer, R.N., M.S.N.
Nurse Practitioner, Ambulatory Care Unit,
Veterans Administration Hospital,
Tucson, Arizona

Lois E. Prosser, R.N., M.S.
Associate Professor of Community Health Nursing,
College of Nursing, The University of Arizona,
Tucson, Arizona

Arlene M. Putt, R.N., Ed. D.
Professor of Nursing,
College of Nursing, The University of Arizona,
Tuscon, Arizona

Sally A. Santmyer, R.N., M.S., P.C.N.S.
Clinical Nurse Specialist, Nursing Service,
St. Mary's Hospital,
Richmond, Virginia

Kathryn E. Smallwood, R.N., B.S.N.
Staff Nurse, Emergency Department,
City of Memphis Hospitals,
Memphis, Tennessee

Judith Twitchell, R.N., M.S.
Nursing/Patient Education Coordinator, Nursing Service,
Valley View Hospital and Medical Center,
Denver, Colorado

Contents

Introduction to General Systems Theory

1

Arlene M. Putt

The Development of General Systems Theory

According to Ashby [1], there exists a science of wholes, with its own laws, methods, logic, and mathematics. This science is known as general systems theory. Boulding [2, p. 1] has referred to general systems theory as the "skeleton of science, a body of theoretical constructs which will serve to express general relationships of the empirical world." Klir [4, p. 1] phrased the idea as follows: "*General systems theory* in the broadest sense refers to a collection of general concepts, principles, tools, problems, methods, and techniques associated with systems." As von Bertalanffy [9, p. 30] described it, "General systems theory then consists of the scientific exploration of 'wholes' and 'wholeness'... the interdisciplinary nature of concepts, models, and principles applying to 'systems' provides a possible approach toward the unification of science."

The concepts for general systems theory were first made public in the late 1920s, and the ideas were formalized in 1954 with the establishment of the Society for General Systems Research, an affiliate of the American Association for the Advancement of Science. In addition, a task force was formed on "general systems theory and psychiatry" in the American Psychiatric Association. In the intervening time, systems thinking has traversed the theoretical sphere to the areas of applied science, becoming the focal point for scientific thought. As Ashby [1, p. 95] said, "Systems theory is essentially a demand that we treat systems as wholes composed of related parts, between which interaction occurs to a major degree." By providing some unification to scientific thought, general systems theory facilitates interdisciplinary endeavors. As Weinberg [11, p. 104] phrased it, "the general systems theorists' chosen task [is] to understand the simplifying assumptions of a science – those assumptions which delimit its field of application and magnify its power of prediction." Weinberg continued to explain that learning and scientific progress evolve from observations that reveal invariant truths about the topics under study.

Orchard [6] has characterized systems theory as divided into four types. Type I theories Orchard identified as *specific theories* dealing with particular interests within a single discipline and are of interest only to the discipline involved. *Generalized systems theories,* type II theories, are generalizations derived from overlapping type I theories, and as such are isomorphic in nature. At the level of type III, theories reflect fundamental characteristics of all systems and contain general principles of methodology. Orchard termed type III theories *general systems theories.* At Orchard's highest level of generalization occur theories with decreasing content; these are the type IV theories – *mathematical theories of systems* – more infinite abstractions of type III general systems theory.

Exploration of the relationships between sets of two of the four levels of theory leads periodically to further integration with increased content and broadened application. Therefore, as described by Weinberg [11, p. 138], *general systems theory* is a set of "ways of looking at the world." This view of the world aids man in his understanding of his relationship with his universe.

The Nature of Systems

To explore general systems theory as applied to nursing, one must first understand the nature of systems. Klir [4] described a system as an arrangement of component parts so interrelated as to form a whole. Hall and Fagen [3] defined a system as a set of relationships between objects and their properties or attributes. Attributes may be common to a number of objects which are the components of a system. Bonds or relationships tie the system together, making it a functioning unit. Surrounding every system is an environment that is either open or closed to other influences. The surrounding environment contains sets of objects that affect both the system and the changes that may occur within it.

The properties or attributes that systems demonstrate may be described as follows.

1. **Nature.** According to Pierce [7], systems can be conceptual or real. Conceptual systems are composed of words, constructs, or symbols. In contrast, real systems are physical entities that occur naturally or are derived by man.
2. **Structure.** The structure of a system refers to the arrangement of the component parts.
3. **Process.** Process refers to the functioning of the system with the exchanges of energy, matter, and information that take place.
4. **Order.** Löfgren [5] noted that the word system is frequently used as a synonym for order. In the concept of order, the idea of hierarchy or ranking is implied. All systems are arranged into an interlocking interacting hierarchy of order based upon size ranging from the microscopic to the cosmic. For the purpose of analysis, any system can be subdivided into subsystems and its parts manipulated.
5. **Wholeness of the unit with interdependence of variables.** In systems, objects and their properties, called *attributes,* are frequently interrelated so that a change in one part can affect the total system. Weinberg [11] explained that

independence of variables, in which the behavior of one variable cannot be predicted from the behavior of other variables and the action in one part does not affect the total functioning, could occur only in a closed system. Therefore, Weinberg concluded that truly independent variables do not exist. All systems have a relative wholeness or else the system could not function as a unit.

6. **Exchange of energies.** A system exists to serve a function. Functioning requires that energy be shared or changed in form and location. Energy exchanges occur at rates varying from extremely slow to very rapid, with some of the exchanges reversible and other exchanges irreversible. By absorbing energy, all systems have potential for increasing their order or complexity. Contrarily, all systems have potential for increasing their disorder or disruption through the dissipation of energy.
7. **Change with time.** Most real systems change with time, either decaying in time or growing toward a higher level of organization. With increasing complexity comes increasing centralization. As complexity increases, one part must emerge as the controlling unit of the system. Systems in interaction with their environment tend to move toward greater specialization of function.
8. **Degree of openness.** Systems may be either open or closed to their environments. Open systems freely exchange energies in the form of materials or information, or both, with their environments. Contrastingly, a closed system is sealed off from its environment and there is no interaction with the surroundings. An open system may become closed if the exchange of materials, information, or energies is halted. In like manner, a closed system may become open if an exchange of energies begins between the system and its enveloping environment.
9. **Degree of stability.** Systems may be adaptive or stable. Adaptation is related to learning and to evolution, and it occurs in degrees; however, flexibility can be interpreted as a measure of instability in the system. Likewise, stability of a system can be equated with nonadaptation. Rapoport [8] described stability as the tendency of a system to return to its equilibrium, and instability as the tendency to depart from equilibrium when the system is disturbed.
10. **Self-correction via feedback.** To provide for self-correction, systems frequently contain a feedback loop designed so that a small portion of the output or information is returned to the system, providing additional information that the system can use to adjust its output.
11. **Isomorphism.** Von Bertalanffy [10] noted that totally different systems frequently have similar components. This useful attribute of systems permits transference of knowledge regarding the functioning of one system to the understanding of another system that may exist in a vastly different but parallel context.

"A system, then," von Bertalanffy [10, p. 31] summarized, "is a conceptual analogue of certain rather universal traits of observed entities." These entities are sets of elements related among themselves and to their environments. The sets have order and exchange energies.

Because systems have "rather universal traits," the study of such traits permits certain generalizations to be made regarding the structure and functioning of systems. Making such generalizations or transferring understandings can facilitate the study of diverse realities. Therefore, a study of systems is worthwhile because of the broad applicability of the principles of systems theory to many fields of endeavor, including nursing.

Basic Concepts of General Systems Theory

In living systems, defined by von Bertalanffy [9] as hierarchically organized open systems maintaining themselves or developing toward a steady state, the basic concepts of general systems theory are those of *entropy, evolution, equifinality, multifinality, feedback,* and *control of subsystems.*

Underlying the concept of *entropy* in general systems theory is the second law of thermodynamics, which states that an isolated system, in essence a system closed to its environment, if left to itself, will tend to increase its disorganization, its randomness. This tendency to increasing randomness by dissipation of energy is termed *entropy.* According to general systems theory, the process of entropy is universal, a force existing in open systems of the social sciences as well as in the closed systems of physical sciences where the process was first noted. If carried to its theoretical end, the final effect of entropy is randomness to infinity, leading to the deterioration and death of the system. The concept of entropy has multiple applications in diverse endeavors.

Some theorists have termed the counterforce to entropy to be negative entropy or negentropy, a double-negative concept [8, 12]. This author prefers a positive term for a positive force; that term is *evolution.* According to the definition in *The Random House Dictionary of the English Language* (College Edition, 1968) evolution means increasing complexity and higher organization. The process of absorbing energy can lead the system to increased organization and complexity, termed *evolution.* Evolution can also imply an active process that requires some expenditure of energy to maintain itself at the present level. Wiener [12] reasoned that information represents a measure of organization. As such, information can be a positive factor, a manifestation of energy exchange in the process of evolution.

Equifinality, another concept in general systems theory, implies that an end or characteristic state can be reached in all open systems independent of the starting point. Equifinality, then, indicates the sameness of the end derived from varying approaches and varying previous existing states.

In opposition to equifinality is the concept of *multifinality,* another idea in which the end state has various possibilities. In multifinal situations, the means selected affect the outcome so that the choice of means must rest upon reason to ensure the desired outcome.

The model of opposing forces of entropy and evolution, coupled with equifinality or with multifinality, can explain many kinds of dynamic vital processes. Evolution of higher forms of life and more complex societies is the result of the constant interplay of entropy and evolution within open systems.

One more concept germane to general systems theory is the concept of *feedback.* Through this mechanism, a small portion of the output of the system is redirected in a backward direction as additional input to allow the system to correct further output. This feedback loop allows systems to be self-directing.

A final characteristic of general systems conceptualization is the idea of the *control of subsystems.* Through increasing centralization, one part of the system must emerge as the controlling unit capable of integrating the actions of the subparts of the system. This process allows for integration of the total organism and the possibility of unified action.

References

1. Ashby, W. R. Systems and Their Informational Measures. In G. J. Klir (Ed.), *Trends in General Systems Theory.* New York: John Wiley & Sons, 1972.
2. Boulding, K. General Systems Theory: The Skeleton of Science. In W. Buckley (Ed.), *Modern Systems Research for the Behavioral Scientist.* Chicago: Aldine Publishing, 1968.
3. Hall, A. D., and Fagen, R. E. Definition of a System. In W. Buckley (Ed.), *Modern Systems Research for the Behavioral Scientist.* Chicago: Aldine Publishing, 1968.
4. Klir, G. J. Preview: The Polyphonic General Systems Theory. In G. J. Klir (Ed.), *Trends in General Systems Theory.* New York: John Wiley & Sons, 1972.
5. Löfgren, L. Relative Explanations of Systems. In G. J. Klir (Ed.), *Trends in General Systems Theory.* New York: John Wiley & Sons, 1972.
6. Orchard, R. A. On An Approach to General Systems Theory. In G. J. Klir (Ed.), *Trends in General Systems Theory.* New York: John Wiley & Sons, 1972.
7. Pierce, L. Usefulness of a systems approach for problem conceptualization and investigation. *Nurs. Res.* 21:507, 1972.
8. Rapoport, A. The Uses of Mathematical Isomorphism in General Systems Theory. In G. J. Klir (Ed.), *Trends in General Systems Theory.* New York: John Wiley & Sons, 1972.
9. von Bertalanffy, L. General System Theory: A Critical Review. In W. Buckley (Ed.), *Modern Systems Research for the Behavioral Scientist.* Chicago: Aldine Publishing, 1968.
10. von Bertalanffy, L. The History and Status of General Systems Theory. In G. J. Klir (Ed.), *Trends in General Systems Theory.* New York: John Wiley & Sons, 1972.
11. Weinberg, G. M. A Computer Approach to General Systems Theory. In G. J. Klir (Ed.), *Trends in General Systems Theory.* New York: John Wiley & Sons, 1972.
12. Wiener, N. Cybernetics in History. In W. Buckley (Ed.), *Modern Systems Research for the Behavioral Scientist.* Chicago: Aldine Publishing, 1968.

Theory Structure and Development 2

I. The Structure of Theory

Arlene M. Putt

According to Jacox [3], "The purpose of a scientific theory is to describe, explain and predict a part of the empirical world." The same purpose can be ascribed to nursing theory. Although it is in varying stages of development, nursing theory does exist and must continue to exist, or else, to paraphrase Pasteur, nursing practice will become routines merely born of habit.

To identify nursing theory in its various stages of development, it is necessary to understand the component parts of theory and the steps through which theory is developed. According to Dickoff, James, and Weidenbach [2], theory begins in practice, is refined through research, and then is returned to practice. After elaboration on their work as well as on the work of Jacox [3], the steps of theory development can be seen as follows.

1. **Criticism or faultfinding.** Criticism is the result of concern. One does not bother to criticize something about which one is indifferent. A criticism serves to articulate the belief that something is amiss and brings to awareness one or more salient features of the situation. Frequently, the process is aborted at this initial step, and movement to a more constructive reaction is never achieved.
2. **Statement of the problem.** A desire to improve the situation results in a delineation of the problem with a refinement of the criticism to the point of being articulate about the defect in the situation. Delineation of the problem involves the following steps.
   a. **Concept identification.** A concept is a term that has been given an operational meaning. Key ideas, thoughts, and words in a problem become concepts that require further exploration and delineation to create a precise meaning. Concepts, according to Abbey [1], are individual, idiosyncratic impressions with distinguishing attributes that can be related within a framework. Thus, attributes of concepts can be divided into categories

such as values, number, form, dominance, size, and color. Jacox [3, p. 5] described concepts as the "abstract representations of reality" that "indicate the subject matter of theory." Constructs are more complex entities "constructed of concepts that are directly or indirectly observable" [3, p. 6].

b. **Proposition or principle formation.** A statement of generalization called a proposition or principle relates two or more concepts or facts, thereby serving to reduce the complexity of the problem [1].

3. **Theory construction.** The product of linking propositions or principles deductively is theory, a conceptual framework designed to show interrelationships. Theory construction, then, is the systematic hierarchical arrangement of propositions. Rules of generalization provide one type of guide for prediction of outcome and thus serve as a guide to action; however, Dickoff, James, and Weidenbach [2] identified theory as existing on four levels, namely: factor-isolating, factor-relating, situation-relating, and situation-producing theory; the last-named is also called prescriptive theory. Each of these levels of theory presupposes lower-level supporting theories. Prescriptive theory has the essential ingredients of a justifiable goal, a prescription of activity to achieve that goal, and a number of component parts, which are defined as follows:
   a. Agency: the performer of the action
   b. Patiency: the recipient of the action
   c. Framework: the context of the situation
   d. Terminus: the end point of the activity
   e. Procedure: the protocol for the activity
   f. Dynamics: the type and amount of energy utilized

   These terms are further clarified in the glossary.

   By the systematic organization of propositions about these attributes, prescriptive theory may be constructed, utilizing the processes of induction and deduction. To clarify the role of theory in nursing practice further, Jacox [3] stated that theory in one field may be utilized as a model in another field if the elements of the theory behave in the same way in both fields. Kaplan [4] identified an empirical theoretical continuum to theory such that any given theory can be located at some point on the continuum where it will have some reference to reality. Theory may be clarified with the use of models as discussed by Riehl and Roy [5].
4. **Validation of theory.** Once developed, theory can serve as a guide for:
   a. Collection of facts
   b. Search for new knowledge
   c. Explanation of the nature of the phenomena being studied
   d. Further action

The professional nurse can put theory to the same uses. She can and should develop and use theory to collect facts, seek new knowledge, explain phenomena, and direct nursing action. With such use of theory, the nurse functions at a professional level, as opposed to becoming the heir to routines born of habit; however, theory can be taken one more step. By testing theory in practice, theory can be validated and then be considered to be doctrine or essential truth. Validation of theory is the end point of theory and the beginning of scientific fact that then can be utilized in nursing practice.

In summary, then, the steps in the development of theory are as follows:

1. Articulation of criticism
2. Statement of the problem through
   a. Identification of the concepts involved
   b. Formation of propositions or principles from two or more concepts
3. Construction of theory by relating concepts and propositions in hierarchical order
4. Testing theory in practice to validate it and produce a fact which can be incorporated into nursing practice as evidence of a scientific basis for nursing action

Based then on an understanding of how theory is developed, the purpose of this book is to show how general systems theory can be applied to nursing problems to provide a reasoned basis for the selected actions. In this way, general systems theory can be applied to validate nursing actions.

References

1. Abbey, J. C. Concepts and Principles. In J. Smith (Ed.), *Five Years of Cooperation To Improve Curricula in Western Schools of Nursing.* Boulder, Colo.: Western Interstate Commission for Higher Education, 1972. P. 6.
2. Dickoff, J., James, P., and Weidenbach, E. Theory in a practice discipline: Part I. *Nurs. Res.* 17:415, 1968.
3. Jacox, A. Theory construction in nursing: An overview. *Nurs. Res.* 23:4, 1974.
4. Kaplan, A. *The Conduct of Inquiry.* San Francisco, Calif.: Chandler & Sharp, 1964.
5. Riehl, J. P., and Roy, C., Sr. *Conceptual Models for Nursing Practice.* New York: Appleton-Century-Crofts, 1974.

II. Concepts and Principles

June C. Abbey

Concepts are traditionally defined as a class of stimuli having common characteristics, but in reality they are impressions, individual and idiosyncratic, that cause factors to be related in a framework – a framework into which the person

Reprinted from J. Smith (Ed.), *Improvement of Curricula in Schools of Nursing Through Selection and Application of Care Concepts of Nursing: An Interim Report.* Boulder, Colo.: Western Interstate Commission for Higher Education, 1970.

presses experience, interpretation, and emotional components, so that the very stimuli are distorted. For instance, think of a butterfly. A butterfly is a concept and, although we are in overall accord that we are talking about an insect that flies, it is impossible without much more discussion and many more adjectives to arrive at any consensus of which butterfly, what it looks like, its size, ability to fly, or an infinitesimal variety of other attributes. Still, we can say "butterfly" and each of us will be able to begin to communicate, to think together, and to develop our own particular knowledge of this elusive insect. Thus, a concept may or may not be congruent with personal experience. It is also apparent that the general concept or "class of stimuli with common characteristics" is in fact different from a particular concept. The distinguishing features are called attributes.

Attributes have been divided into categories of values, number, dominance, and form or shape. Oddly, but not surprisingly, people incorporate these attributes into their conceptual learning at different rates. Some features of the concept are more dominant or more obvious than others. Archer [1] finds that size or shape dominates the *value* of color or of number differentiation. Therefore, if one is teaching a skill such as the use of syringes, the differences in size should be coupled with the differences in use. Rather than presenting a multiplicity of various sizes, a 2-ml. and a tubercular luer are given to the student to manipulate. The quantities of solution are compared and contrasted, and attention called to the markings. Color follows size in *dominance* [20]. Colors, therefore, become conceptual, integrating signposts. Again, contrast and comparison aid in the recall of color with subsequent accurate conceptualization.

Number is peculiarly susceptible to being taught as a concept because this attribute varies with familiarity, context, and *perception* of importance to the conceptualizer. To conserve time, the individual may reduce the number to which he attends [6], or under stress he may be unable to perceive the "how manys." The expert is empowered by his familiarity to generalize from his existing conceptual framework to incorporate the novel; the amateur, not knowing what is unusual and lacking a concept of structure, may not be able to formulate the overall picture or pattern-idea.

Wallace [21] states: "When defining concepts, teachers resort to emphases to make obscure attributes obvious." It is important also to note that unless this emphasis is provided, and if any attributes are missed, the concept will be incomplete. Additional building onto the conceptual framework will be skewed by the omission, and the success of concept incorporation into care settings will be unpredictable.

Types of Concepts and Principles

Concepts

Concepts can be of a conjunctive, disjunctive, or relational nature. In *conjunctive* concepts, several similar values are jointly present. For example, green circles are conjunctive in number, color, and shape (form). Conjunctive concepts are easier to teach than disjunctive concepts because the attributes are additive. Hence, similarity promotes recall. The pale patient suggests to the observer a number of signs and symptoms associated with an ashen or anemic face, such as fatigue, cold, weakness, etc. *Disjunctive* concepts are those in which one or more attributes do not match. An example would be two figures and two circles of the same color. Both form and numbers can differ, while the color value remains the same. Six different arrangements can be made. If one were to increase the factors to three green figures and three green circles, there are 81 possible permutations. Disjunctive concepts are therefore more difficult to learn because of the arbitrary equilibration of the attributes. They are also more difficult to teach because contrast must be made on each in increment and combination of increments. *Relational* concepts clearly define the relationship between two attributes such as distance and direction [8]. Note both have the same attributes; i.e., distance specifies the relationship between two spots. In nursing, one might sum these up as conjunctive or comparative concepts, disjunctive or contrasting concepts, and relational or cause-and-effect concepts.

Principles

The statement of relationship between two or more concepts becomes a rule for generalization and is called a *principle* [11]. For example, if the patient hemorrhages and the blood volume decreases, the heart rate will increase. The relationship between the concepts of hemorrhage, blood volume, and heart rate is combined into an if-then principle.

Use of Concepts and Principles

Concepts and principles reduce the complexity of the environment. By extracting the essence of this idea, the learner can manipulate the factors and utilize the concept in novel situations. The simplification of the entire learning construct into a conceptual hierarchy demands insight as well as knowledge of the subject. Truly, as Archer states, the "...highest level of sophistication exists when all individuals can with ease decrease complexity while appreciating subtle differences of the material."[2]

Through the use of concepts and principles, objects of the world are identified or placed in a class, and complexity is hence lessened. Identification is never absent from behavior. First learning, according to Piaget, is directed toward the concrete objects within the immediate environment. The child between the ages of 7 and 11 needs the physical attributes of a concept for identification. When a gap occurs, the organization is isolated and the concept is unrelated to the real world. While requiring abstract thought and available memory manipulation, the schemata exist in 11-year-olds only as a real object or situation. The child thinks concretely but can bring to bear memory or past experiences. The preschool child, by contrast, is limited in the use of his concepts to current experience [8]. The adult builds upon experience, maneuvers his recall, but also uses propositions of if-then to formulate new concepts and string ideas into principles.

The ability to identify is the basis for *entering behavior* into the situation. Entering behavior is defined as the abilities and levels of knowledge that a student brings to the learning situation. The learner attends, classifies, and identifies the new. The teacher formulates the class content between entering-behavior levels and the course objectives. Concepts, therefore, enable the student to progress through the discipline by modifying and increasing his own knowledge. These patterns and frameworks can, if not subjected to constant revision, become resistant to change. Bayley [4] feels that "increased age means increased resistance to breaking old patterns of organized knowledge." Biological studies by Guilford on learning ability, however, reveal that the depth of the cortex continues to grow until the age of 45 and that the posterior cortex apparently is the area for abstracting "the common properties of things" [14], clearly disputing Bayley [4]. It would seem that learning is not primarily limited by physiological aging but by past learning patterns.

In nursing, the use of concept and principle gives concerted direction for activity. Nursing is a doing, decision-making profession. Placement of a gestalt into the proper class of concepts and principles can promote optimum patient care. A case in point would be a patient with a paradoxical pulse. From the rather routine assessment of taking a blood pressure reading, the nurse could determine that the heart had insufficient force to pump against the increased intrathoracic pressure accompanying normal breathing. During this interim, back pressure into the portal circulation would occur; therefore, the patient might be subject to hepatic dysfunction and have difficulty with immune body formation. The resultant nursing measure of protection from sources of secondary infection is the compilation and relationship of the foregoing conceptual framework.

Concepts and principles facilitate instruction because, once labeled with a specific word, they are aroused to immediate recall and the teacher does not need to cover old territory. Gagne [10, p. 139] states that the "great value of concepts is that they refer to concrete environment." If this is true, concepts could become a formidable obstacle to instruction if the student's grasp is inadequate, and hence no relationship can exist with the environment. If stereotyped, the concept could then be rigid, inaccurate, and impervious to experience [16].

Teaching Concepts

A change in the behavior of the student is evidence that a concept has been learned. Such a performance change shows the differences made on entering behavior by the acquisition of the new concept. The teacher must, therefore, be able to describe the expected activities of the learner after the concept has been learned. This terminal performance description correctly identifies behavioral examples of the newly acquired concept and is written by the instructor prior to teaching the learner. The statement is then shared with the student. In addition to providing means for assessment and determining the need for further instruction, it promotes student assessment and facilitates the ability to evaluate when learning is complete. Such involvement of the student in self-assessment also affords internal or self-reinforcement.

Complex concepts consist of a multiplicity of attributes. To facilitate learning, the most important characteristics are made dominant and emphasized. Attributes are grouped conjunctively. Verbal mediators (words of explanation), labels, and sources of identification promote learning, although some studies dispute the myth that even young children learn concepts best through intensive instructional guidance [23, 24]. The research of Huttenlocher [15] shows that students learn best from both positive and negative examples of the concept. This comparison and contrast provide additional sources for discrimination and generalization. As mentioned previously, negative examples are the most difficult to learn because they are extraneous to the pattern and must be remembered [5].

Teachers of nursing characteristically present real examples of the clinical setting. The student readily recognizes the relationship of the concept to the patient. Care should be exercised in the selection of the examples. The teacher must experiment with the concepts to discover the places where there may be student hang-ups or difficulties. An incomplete concept is a nonapplicable concept and hence unrelated to the experiential realism necessary for future integration.

Nursing lends itself to the developmental schemata of concept formation by its very nonstatic nature, in which each task leads to the next. Instructors can easily create a focus condition of two examples of a concept occurring simultaneously. Later, recall of either incites memory of the other, and the concept is reinforced.

Students learn concepts first by identification. The concept is recognized as part of a given experimental milieu of the classroom, conference, or clinical setting. Generally, if questioned, the entire situation in which the conceptualization happened can be remembered and the concept described, or if described by the teacher, recognized by the student. Naming or labeling occurs next, as the learner codifies the pattern for instant use. This identification process can be used by the teacher to check learning and provide an opportunity for reinforcement. Often students can identify but not define a concept. While this capacity is useful to the instructor for assessment of topical content, the learner cannot manipulate the concept easily enough for use in patient teaching or clinical application. Often, special training is necessary to help the student hurdle the barrier of identification, definition, and manipulation to application.

Reinforcement and Concept Learning

Research shows conclusively that reinforcement is an effective technique in promoting concept learning. In addition to providing informational feedback, more difficult concepts can be learned with fewer examples if the reinforcement feedback is intense [21] and related to the experiential situation. By contrast, delayed reinforcement, postponed as little as 40 minutes, lessens concept learning [19], and negative verbal feedback will decrease the hypothesis-testing device of making guesses about a concept. The educator must be aware that such exploration is necessary for the internalization and definition of the concept and related principles by the student. Therefore, the use of such negative feedback dictates caution.

Much has been said about the influence of watching others model behavior on the learner's performance. Popular television programming is a battleground of the pros and cons of the effects on children of watching violence. Studies show definitely, however, that viewing punitive feedback for an action causes the child to avoid that particular activity [3]. If the response frequency is thereby diminished, there will be fewer opportunities for any type of reinforcement, and the concept will take longer to learn. A case in point would be punitive correction of one student witnessed by another. A classmate makes a medication error for which he is reprimanded. The witness becomes reluctant to give medication and therefore takes advantage of fewer opportunities to practice. The teacher will also find fewer chances to reinforce the second student's performance and to promote concept learning.

Learning is also affected by the consistency of reinforcement. Rhine and Silum [17] found that when feedback was always given and was 100 percent in accord with the concept, the ability to learn concepts increased. Carpenter [7] had previously shown that partial reinforcement was not as effective as consistent feedback. Scientific concepts present an additional aspect of consistency when, if the mode of response required shifts from mathematical to verbal expression, a diminished ability to express the concept is evidenced [22]. In nursing education, the converse is more often true, with the student being able to state the concept verbally but having great difficulty in using mathematical formulation and numerical relationships.

Teaching Principles

The teaching of principles follows the general format of teaching concepts. Terminal performance, or what the student will be able to do after learning takes place, should be described and stated as behavioral objectives. Entering behavior is then assessed and the difference between the two studied to determine what concepts or principles are necessary for recall in order to learn the new principle. The questions revolve around "What does the learner need to know in order to grasp this principle?" As the component concepts emerge, a hierarchy or "structure of organized knowledge about the topic" [9, 12, 13] develops, which gives the teacher the proper order of the concepts to assist the student in recall and combination of concepts into the new principle.

After becoming aware of the principle the student should be required to demonstrate and to state the principle fully. Opportunity to use the newly acquired principle in a novel situation affords verification that learning has actually taken place and that the student has not simply combined rote factors without true integration. The last two steps are the provision of time for practice and reinforcement in as great a variety of settings as possible.

The evaluation process includes both the teaching schemata and the student performance. Each of these is subjected to rigorous scrutiny because poor teaching or inadequate learning can contribute equally to minimal performance. Principles built of incomplete concepts are incomplete principles, limited in application and difficult for the student to integrate. Instead of offering bridges to future learning, their use is confined to experiential testing and tested situations. When teaching simple-to-complex principles, the instructor must study the content contained in a principle for difficult areas (1) prior to student exposure and (2) following the student's learning to discover what retards assimilation in any particular area.

One common error in evaluating the learning of principles may relate to the time it takes for integration. Recent studies [18] show that the rate of learning is similar between the slow learner and the fast learner once a basic "getting ready to learn" pattern occurs; however, the so-called better student starts more quickly and, therefore, can learn for a longer period in a prescribed length of time. The slow student's learning curve, while depicting a longer "lead-time" (getting ready to learn), has an identical slope and height. While Samuels' research [18] was done on reading and arithmetic tasks in elementary schools, his follow-up studies on these students suggest that their learning patterns persist throughout high school in both the natural and social sciences. In teaching principles, therefore, evaluation of lead-time for acquisition might well be incorporated into individualized clinical teaching. For instance, setting might contribute to lead-time and be held relatively stable when new learning tasks are introduced.

The teaching of principles demands constant evaluation both by the learner and the teacher. If the expected end performance is formally stated in written form, the instructor can determine with the learner the degree and extent of learning. Comparison and contrast are possible. Principles can once more be broken down to their original component concepts and be reassembled into different, more applicable principles. From this process, relevance constantly tests new ideas for improvement to be incorporated into future learning situations.

Concepts are fundamental tools for learning and instruments for recall, and, when incorporated into principles, become complex servo-dynamic mechanisms (see Glossary) for application and integration. Factors of an instructor's teaching, composites of a student's learning, these frameworks become the basis of intellectual prowess. Even more important, as the directors of perception, concepts determine an individual's very behavior. Here then are increments of values, of ethics; here the learner's system of servo-dynamic mechanisms can be influenced, and herein lies the power of teaching.

References

1. Archer, E. J. Concept identification as a function of obviousness of relevant and irrelevant information. *J. Exp. Psychol.* (Gen.) 63:616, 1962.

2. Archer, E. J. The Psychological Nature of Concepts. In H. J. Klausmeier and C. W. Harris (Eds.), *Analyses of Concept Learning.* New York: Academic Press, 1966.
3. Bandura, A., Grusec, J. E., and Menlove, F. L. Vicarious extinction of avoidance behavior. *J. Pers. Soc. Psychol.* 5:16, 1967.
4. Bayley, N. Learning in Adulthood: The Role of Intelligence. In H. J. Klausmeier and C. W. Harris (Eds.), *Analyses of Concept Learning.* New York: Academic Press, 1966.
5. Braley, L. Strategy selection and negative instances in concept learning. *J. Educ. Psychol.* 54:154, 1963.
6. Bruner, J. S., Goodnow, J. J., and Austin, G. A. *A Study of Thinking.* New York: John Wiley & Sons, 1956.
7. Carpenter, F. Conceptualization as a function of differential reinforcement. *Sci. Ed.* 38:284, 329, 1954.
8. Carroll, J. B. Words, meanings, and concepts. *Harv. Educ. Rev.* 34:178, 1964.
9. Gagne, R. M. The acquisition of knowledge. *Psychol. Rev.* 69:355, 1962.
10. Gagne, R. M. *Conditions of Learning.* New York: Holt, Rinehart & Winston, 1965.
11. Gagne, R. M. The Learning of Principles. In H. J. Klausmeier and C. W. Harris (Eds.), *Analyses of Concept Learning.* New York: Academic Press, 1966.
12. Gagne, R. M., and Bessler, O. C. Study of retention in some topics of elementary nonmetric geometry. *J. Educ. Psychol.* (Gen.) 54:123, 1963.
13. Gagne, R. M., and Brown, L. T. Some factors in programming of conceptual learning. *J. Exp. Psychol.* 62:313, 1961.
14. Guilford, J. P. *The Nature of Human Intelligence.* New York: McGraw-Hill, 1967.
15. Huttenlocher, J. Some effects of negative instances in the formation of simple concepts. *Psychol. Rep.* 11:35, 1962.
16. McDonald, F. J. *Educational Psychology.* (2d ed.). Belmont, Calif.: Wadsworth Publishing Co., 1965.
17. Rhine, R. J., and Silun, B. A. Acquisition and change of a concept attitude as a function of consistency of reinforcement. *J. Exp. Psychol.* 55:524, 1958.
18. Samuels, S. J. Learning Curves: A Family of Curves. Unpublished manuscript, 1969.
19. Sax, G. Concept acquisitions as a function of differing schedules and delays of reinforcement. *J. Educ. Psychol.* (Gen.) 51:32, 1960.
20. Sechrest, L., and Kaas, J. S. Concept difficulty as a function of stimulus similarity. *J. Educ. Psychol.* (Gen.) 56:327, 1965.
21. Wallace, J. Concept dominance, type of feedback, and intensity of feedback as related to concept attainment. *J. Educ. Psychol.* (Gen.) 55:158, 1964.
22. Wilder, N., and Green, D. R. Expressions of concepts through writing and drawing: Effects of shifting medium. *J. Educ. Psychol.* (Gen.) 54:202, 1963.
23. Wittrock, M. C. Verbal stimuli in concept formation: Learning by discovery. *J. Educ. Psychol.* (Gen.) 64:183, 1963.
24. Wittrock, M. C., Keisler, E., and Stern, C. Verbal cues in concept identification. *J. Educ. Psychol.* (Gen.) 55:195, 1964.

Living Systems in Interlocking Hierarchy

3

Arlene M. Putt

Living systems, open to their environment, freely interchanging energy and information with the surrounding matter, maintaining themselves and seeking a steady state, exist in an interlocking hierarchy of size from cosmic to microscopic.

The largest living system that can be visualized with certainty is the planet earth, with its billions of inhabitants of varying orders and species. A living system of a larger order may exist within the universe, but to date no proof of such a system has been found. For the purposes of this book, the earth, then, can be considered as a biomass that conforms to the present limit of size of a living system.

The earth contains subsystems of living things that abide in the fundamental planetary subdivisions of land and water. While the sky does contain living things at times, the origin of life is either on the land or in the fresh or salt water. The waters of the earth are divided into subsystems of oceans. Smaller subdivisions are known as seas, gulfs, bays, and lakes, all fed by various rivers and streams coursing over the land. The land is basically divided into five continents which are again subdivided by some natural boundaries such as mountains, lakes, rivers, seas, and oceans. Man, a creature capable of changing the face and destiny of the entire world, has gone further and arbitrarily created land divisions on the various continents, calling these subdivisions countries. Furthermore, each of the countries is divided into regions, states, counties, districts, and cities; the next lower divisions are smaller units – towns and villages. In all these arbitrary planetary divisions is man, collectively in kinship groups and in groups of unrelated individuals.

While systems of mankind have been considered in decreasing order of magnitude, the pattern of social development has been one of increasing complexity ranging from two individuals, a male and a female, uniting to form a family, and with other families nearby, forming villages, towns, cities, districts, states, and countries. Finally, the countries have united as United Nations. To this point, the frame of reference has been sociological.

When man, his immediate family, and their interaction with neighborhood groupings is considered, the reference becomes psychological. A single individual's perception and reaction to any other individual is a set of unique systems, only part of which may have parallels in other situations.

When the search for systems enters man himself, the realm of physiological entities has been reached. Ferguson [2] described man, singularly or collectively, to be a synthesis of component parts of subsystems. According to Milsum [3], the first level subsystem within man is that of physiological organs such as the respiratory tract with its lungs and the circulatory system with its heart and other attending parts. Basic to each organ are several layers of differentiated structures called tissues composed of rows of similarly designed cells. These layered rows of cells serve some specialized purpose such as secretion or protection. Smaller than a tissue is the cell, considered the ultimate small but complete functioning unit; however, the cell is not a unified structure but is composed of many specialized subunits, each serving a specific function in the scheme of life. Subunits of cells include nuclei, mitochondria, Golgi complexes, and other identifiable entities.

Man, then, is an independently functioning organism, a result of the complex synergistic arrangement of millions of cells through which one can visualize the evolution toward increasing complexity. Just as man himself evolves to greater complexity, man, in his relationship with other men, is seeking greater organization and further development with the goal of greater stability through mutually effective interdependence of parts of the system. If the narrow band of atmosphere continues to support the continuing development of man and his social inventions, the process of evolution of man, the organism, and man, the social creature, can continue ad infinitum. Man, the physiological organism, as explained by Birdwhistell [1], cannot thrive in the absence of social stimulation. Social interaction or communication has become a system through which human beings have established a predictable continuity of life. As such, communication with other organisms is virtually essential for the continuance of human life. A degree of predictability is the quality upon which life is developed. One system learns to predict what another system is likely to do. If the predictability is not correct, certain stresses and strains develop in the interrelationships of the various systems. By understanding better the hierarchy and predictability of mankind's many interwoven systems, better control and correction of the systems can be developed at any of the many intermediate points along the continuum. Better control of the system is the goal of self-correcting systems.

References

1. Birdwhistell, R. L. *Kinesics and Context.* Philadelphia: University of Pennsylvania Press, 1970.
2. Ferguson, C. K. Concerning the Nature of Human Systems and the Consultant's Role. In W. G. Bennis, K. D. Benne, and R. Chin (Eds.), *The Planning of Change.* New York: Holt, Rinehart & Winston, 1969.
3. Milsum. J. H. The Hierarchical Basis for General Living Systems. In G. J. Klir (Ed.), *Trends in General Systems Theory.* New York: John Wiley & Sons, 1972.

General Systems Theory: A Framework for Nursing

4

I. A General Systems Approach to Nursing

June C. Abbey

Nursing, as an emerging profession, finds itself accosted by numerous dilemmas. The most serious of these seems to be that there is no circumscribed body of content [2]. Since the nurse is between the social worker, the psychologist, the physician, the teacher, and the physical scientist, her proposed body of working knowledge must be integrative. If she is to satisfy her role as determined by society to include care, nurturance, support, and involvement, the nurse must be able to draw on, and use clinically, principles from each of the aforementioned disciplines [7]. We must, therefore, discover what principles are common to each discipline: To what basic structure do these concepts relate? Are these concepts universal to the extent of incorporating the ill individual? Could these ideas be worked into a framework for teaching that would promote a pattern of composite thinking in the student and practitioner?

There are few theoretical overviews in nursing. Outstanding theorists are Johnson [8, 9], Reiter [15], and Orlando [12]. Each theorist tends to give emphasis to her own specialty. Still, if as Bruner [4, p. 31] has stated, "... underlying principles give structure to a subject," nursing must have composite principles. Toward this end, general systems were explored and the concept of open and closed systems was extracted [18, 19, 20]. The principles of energy, entropy, gradients, and disorganization commonly found in the basic sciences contributed additional structure, leaving the social sciences as the enigma. Finally, the idea of the Self of Systems presented itself as the overall design.

Characteristics of Systems

General systems have certain characteristics that are true whenever one defines a system no matter what the discipline. All systems are organized units with a

Reprinted from J. Smith (Ed.), *Improvement of Curricula in Schools of Nursing Through Selection and Application of Care Concepts of Nursing: An Interim Report.* Boulder, Colo.: Western Interstate Commission for Higher Education, 1970.

set of components that mutually react. The system acts as a whole; a dysfunction of a part causes a system disturbance rather than the loss of a single function. Further, into all systems regardless of components and interacting forces, activity can be resolved into an aggregation of feedback circuits such as input, servo-mechanisms, and output [1]. Interestingly, this feedback circuit holds in both physical and biological sciences [11]. These feedback circuits function to control variables; modify reaction by facilitation, inhibition, or dissemination; and direct the overall system toward a goal [17] – the primary goal being the maintenance of an intact system. Forces existing between components and activity of the feedback systems result in strains and stresses. In order to obtain congruency, stress is here defined in the classical manner as "internal reorganization in response to strain" [3, p. 161].

Types of Systems

There are two types of systems, closed systems and open systems. The *closed system* consists of specific variables that react with a predictable outcome. While it is possible to change the number of variables included in a closed system, prediction or a high degree of probability differentiates the closed from the open system. For example, the amount of calcium ions in the blood is dependent upon pH, phosphate, and protein-bound calcium in solution [16]. A change in any one of the components predictably affects the calcium ion concentration in this closed system.

Example: The most graphic and common clinical example, perhaps, is the hyperventilating patient who changes the blood pH toward alkalosis by breathing off excessive amounts of carbon dioxide. The resultant tingling, tremors, and muscle spasms are thought to be caused by the decrease in serum calcium with a subsequent change in membrane permeability and irritability. The age-old treatment of breathing into a paper bag causes retention of carbon dioxide, the serum shifts toward normal, and the calcium ions are released. The patient's symptoms then subside.

By contrast, the *open system* consists of a multiplicity of variables that permits a continuous exchange in an orderly process. The outcome is not predictable because of the infinite number of variables. In addition, closed systems can and do exist within open systems. An example of a closed system within an open system is the withdrawal reflex in response to a painful stimulus.

Example: Usually when one touches something painful, the closed system of fine nerve fiber reception internuncial neurons and ventral gray column cells react by withdrawal in less time than it takes to recount the parts of the system; however, the waitress carrying a hot bowl of soup that drips over onto her arm overrules this closed reflex arc. She integrates the closed system into her open system of response to the total milieu and exerts voluntary control through central nervous system inhibition. The soup remains in the bowl. This is a basis for homeostasis, true, but controlled by the open system. Think of the patient who undergoes a painful dressing and remains motionless.

The proposed model thus enables one to look at any part of the system as through a microscope, focusing with different magnifications at the boundaries of various subsystems, selecting a minute closed system, the overall reorganization of the organism, or the interaction of the Self system with its milieu.

Organisms as Systems

All organisms are open systems that enter into an exchange with their environment. This interaction stimulates the internal components to yield an intrinsic activity to the overall system. The boundaries are dynamic and change in response to stress or strain [18]. A steady state is in reality a disequilibrium of subsystems creating tensions and energy displacement which are in turn available to discharge (react) in response to an external stimulus. Interaction between parts of the system necessitates expenditures of some type(s) of energy.

To summarize, the system may be closed or open and its component parts interact in response to strain or stress. Further activities obey basic laws, and energy is necessary to both types of systems.

Energy

In a study of the basic sciences, two things about energy stand out. The first is that "energy" is defined as an ability or as a force [3]. Despite Einstein's theory, we do not know what energy is in any of its forms. Newton said that it was enough to describe what energy did in various circumstances without attempting to state what it was [10]. The second facet is that energy can change its form; it can be transduced. In other words, we have different forms of energy, each of which can be changed into the other. The concept sounds like magic and is, when one considers what things become possible. For instance, the ionic exchange at the cardiac cell membrane (electrochemical energy) causes the heart to beat (mechanical energy) but also can be picked up via an electrode (electrical energy) to be recorded on either a stylus (electrocardiogram) of a mechanical nature or on an oscilloscope as an electrical waveform radiating light energy [6]; however, this transduction from one form to another is expensive and hence part of the energy is lost to the system.

As aforementioned, the interactions between factors result in strains and stresses that cost the system energy. This tendency toward disorganization resulting from energy loss is called entropy. Such loss can be augmented by increased tensions. The existence of a system, whether closed or open, is dependent upon the replacement of this lost energy.

One of the fundamental laws of energy is that to work against an energy gradient requires greater energy, i.e., to drive uphill or, perhaps more appropriate to homeostasis, in order for membrane potential to be reset after firing, the cell must be intact and able to utilize active transport in order to move the sodium out of the cell back into the extracellular fluid. Ischemic, injured cells with metabolic action cannot do this; therefore, they swell as the H_2O moves in to establish equilibrium. Opposing energy gradients complement each other, if of similar kind but opposing quality, as evidenced by plus and minus charges.

Pertinent to the author's theoretical framework are the following applicable factors about energy: (1) Energy can be transduced. (2) Conversion to another form is expensive because some of the total amount is lost in entropy. (3) Existence of a system, whether closed or open, is dependent upon replacement of this lost energy. (4) To work against an energy gradient requires greater energy, i.e., to drive uphill. (5) Opposing energy gradients complement each other, if of similar kind of opposing quality, as is evidenced by plus and minus charges.

Self System

If all the foregoing rules hold, and there is no apparent reason to doubt the authorities, a system could be called a Self. During the formative state, when components are selecting positions in response to other factors, such as the attractions and repulsions of the energies and masses, the system is identifying Self. In an unstable state, energy loss is high, internal repositioning is great, and the boundaries change shape often. The components attempt to form a stabilizing configuration, but because of entropy, this cannot be maintained. Servo-dynamic mechanisms for Self develop in the shape (or form) of feedback loops that work toward equilibration [14]. Their complexity is determined by the size, number of parts, energy requirements, and function of the system. When adequate development of controls occurs, the open system begins to affirm Self. It is able to withstand strains, to adjust its boundaries, and, in living organisms, to repair or reproduce Self.

Some examples are perhaps in order. A person new to a group generally is somewhat cautious; he listens, "sizes things up," and "gets the lay of the land," thereby using psycho-social servo-dynamic mechanisms to identify Self in this new setting. The next step is to make comments which are more or less probes, such as, "You say you're from L.A.? Well, do you know . . .?" Then, if all goes well the assertive, declarative, manipulative affirmation of Self begins. This is not to imply the sequence is exactly the same in every instance, or to make any statement about duration of time in any of the stages.

Another example is the fetus that begins by identifying physiological systems and Self to such an extent that as a neonate he will reject his mother's Rh-negative blood. Later in life, tissues are so identified with Self that they will only replicate Self or cell groupings of the same structure.

The person who is ill must re-identify Self because he cannot become what he was. New servo-dynamic mechanisms must develop before he can affirm Self (assume independence). It seems reasonable that certain feedback loops will be inappropriate to this new Self, and therefore will of themselves create stress. The sense of balance after a leg amputation is a case in point. New and adjusted relationships must set up. The total Self is a contracted system with diminished mobility and, therefore, a decrease in input. Adjustments of the psychological as well as physiological Self systems are in order. It is unreasonable to expect either to respond in a way rational to the previous system. Frustration is of a high order, fed by both feedback loops; compensation is slow, inaccurate, or even inadequate. Energy is wasted as entropy.

The nurse must now effect an energy transfer from a high-energy source to a low-energy source. If one system, i.e., the patient, desires to gain and the other, i.e., the nurse, to give to the patient, the systems are said to fit. A counter-fit occurs when repulsive forces exist. The art of nursing then becomes one of matching energies in amount, kind, degree, and time.

Energy Transfer Recognized

To facilitate energy transfer, the nurse must ascertain the type that is needed by a system to preserve its Self. In other words, if the psychological Self is entropic as in rage, hysteria, or mania, the nurse in this scheme would accept as much of the energy as she could successfully transduce and give back to the patient in an acceptable state [13]. The remainder she would disseminate (share) as widely as possible to prevent upheaval in her own Self system. Dissemination takes place in today's working world hopefully via ward conferences and/or gripe sessions. Formerly the manic, hysterical, or angry patient was wrapped in cold, wet sheets that absorbed the energy being released as entropy in the form of heat. This caused evaporation of the water and dissipation of the heat-energy. As one would expect from the overall concept, the patient became progressively calmer, and the system was able to reestablish itself.

Entropy energy reaction occurs on some terminal wards where the nursing process is one of constant giving. Here self-protective devices (servo-dynamic mechanisms) occur, such as avoidance of parallel conversations with the patient. A relatively recent innovation is psychiatric help for the staff to compensate for this energy drain.

Open systems can never stand still, or stagnate, but can age. Groups lose their purpose, and the numbers look for new identities to promote continuance. Shifts occur in power foci. The aging person in particular demonstrates this contracting totality [5]. Besides the infirmity of gait and movement, other obvious changes occur with the aged. The extremities become thin and spindly, since the decreased pulmonary function does not allow for wasting energy on misplaced fat. Instead, heat (energy) is conserved by increased adipose tissue around the "belly," which acts as insulation to the vital abdominal organs.

The senses are other systems of Self that contract with aging. Not only does one lose visual accommodation and hence close vision, but also other changes occur in actual reception. The sensors appear to be generally refractive to high frequency or intensity, so hearing thus fails in the high ranges while the low tones continue to be heard. Blues and greens are gradually lost to sight while pinks, lavenders, and yellows become preferred. The aged charily weigh the amount of energy any activity costs against the rewards, which results in still greater contraction of systems; however, deprived sensory systems also make compensatory adjustments. The mind creates illusions, hallucinations, and visions in all forms of deprivation. The aged retreat to their memories, the youth daydream of great deeds. In other words, the nurse must promote energy intake by the overall Self system which can then, by stimulation to other internal subsystems, generate action and responses in the systems called Servo-dynamics Mechanisms and Affirmation of Self.

The entire concept must include interactions of the systems of the patient whether they are psychological, physiological, or his Self system within the systems of his ambient social climate. "Our problem," as Whitehead [21, p. 166] has stated, "is in fact, to fit the world to our perceptions and not our perceptions to the world." The patient's defense mechanisms are servo-dynamic in nature and are purposeful in his system.

To appreciate the interplay fully in dealing with an open system, one must be cognizant of the parts. The general rules extend across disciplines to include stresses, strains, and entropy. Every system impinging on another articulates with and changes the relationship of each. Energy deprivation, be it stimuli (i.e., photons, sound waves) or biochemical input, leads to distortion, compensation, and contraction. The system is then forced to re-identify and develop new servo-dynamic mechanisms before it can affirm itself either by expansion, stability, or replication. Every age responds to these dynamisms. Hopefully, this framework will promote a pattern of composite thinking that will permit generalization from the past, organization for the moment, coupled with true motivation for analysis of patient care.

So in closing, World War II did not open gateways to our understandings of the past; rather, it battered down the floodgates of our future. We in nursing must derive conceptualizations that are of the world – the world of the aftermath of the fission of the atom and the world in which fusion of the vast array of particles of knowledge into a homeostatic systemization is necessary for survival.

References

1. Ashby, W. R. Regulation and Control. In W. Buckley (Ed.), *Modern Systems Research for the Behavioral Scientist.* Chicago: Aldine Publishing, 1968.
2. Berthold, J. S. Symposium on theory development in nursing. *Nurs. Res.* 17:196, 1968.
3. Blackwood, O. H., Kelly, C., and Bell, R. M. *General Physics* (3d ed.). New York and London: John Wiley & Sons, 1963.
4. Bruner, J. S. *The Process of Education.* Cambridge: Harvard University Press, 1960.
5. DeLong, A. J. An Outline of the Environmental Language of the Older Person. Paper presented at the sixth annual meeting and conference of the American Association of Homes for the Aging. Mimeographed. October, 1967.
6. Goldman, M. J. *Principles of Clinical Electrocardiography.* Los Altos, Calif.: Lange Medical Publications, 1967.

7. Greenough, K. Determining standards for nursing care. *Am. J. Nurs.* 17:206, 1968.
8. Johnson, D. E. Philosophy of Nursing. *Nurs. Outlook* 7:198, 1959.
9. Johnson, D. E. Theory in nursing: Borrowed and unique. *Nurs. Res.* 17:206, 1968.
10. Karp, W. Sir Isaac Newton. *Horizon* 10:17, 1968.
11. Kremyanski, V. I. Certain Peculiarities of Organisms as a 'System' from the Point of View of Physics, Cybernetics, and Biology. In W. Buckley (Ed.), *Modern Systems Research for the Behavioral Scientist.* Chicago: Aldine Publishing, 1968.
12. Orlando, I. J. *Dynamic Nurse-Patient Relationships.* New York: G. P. Putnam's Sons, 1961.
13. Ostow, M. The Entropy Concept and Psychic Function. In W. Buckley (Ed.), *Modern Systems Research for the Behavioral Scientist.* Chicago: Aldine Publishing, 1968.
14. Redfield, R. (Ed.). *Levels of Integration in Biological and Social Systems* (Introduction). Lancaster, Pa.: Jacques Catell Press, 1942.
15. Reiter, F. Nurse-clinician. *Am. J. Nurs.* 66:274, 1966.
16. Selkurt, E. E. (Ed.). *Physiology* (2d ed.). Boston: Little, Brown, 1966.
17. von Bekesy, A. G. *Sensory Inhibition.* Princeton: Princeton University Press, 1967.
18. von Bertalanffy, L. *Robots, Men, and Minds.* New York: George Braziller, 1967.
19. von Bertalanffy, L. General Systems Theory and Psychiatry. In *American Handbook of Psychiatry,* Vol. 3. New York: George Braziller, 1968, p. 705.
20. Weiner, N. *The Human Use of Human Beings: Cybernetics and Society.* Garden City, N.Y.: Doubleday, Anchor Press, 1954.
21. Whitehead, A. N. *Aims of Education.* New York: Macmillan, 1959.

II. General Systems Theory: A Guide for Nursing

Arlene M. Putt

According to Brillouin [2, p. 147], "Life cannot be understood without reference to a 'life principle.' The behavior of living organisms is completely different from that of inert matter." Brillouin [2, p. 153] declared that "the entropy content of a living organism is a completely meaningless notion" for it cannot be measured. Raymond [7, p. 160] counterchecked Brillouin's thought by saying, "Although it is quite true that operations for the determination of entropy of living organisms according to current thermodynamic definitions do not exist, it is possible that such operations might be devised . . ."

"Life," wrote Schrödinger [9, p. 143], "seems to be orderly and lawful behavior of matter, not based exclusively on its tendency to go over from order to disorder, but based partly on existing order that is kept up." Raymond [7, p. 170] went on to conceptualize "the use of the concept of entropy as an indication of the state of health of an organism."

At this point, the general systems theory, as developed by von Bertalanffy [11] and explained by Abbey [1], can be related to nursing. Hazzard [3, p. 386] declared "nursing is a system because it consists of elements in interaction." Rogers [8] recognized the interchange of matter and energy between man and his environment as one postulate on which she based her theoretical basis of nursing.

McKay [4] has very aptly described nursing as a biopsychosocial process. As such, the forces of entropy and evolution are involved [6]. In these two forces of entropy and evolution are the ebb and flow of life. This model of opposing forces can explain many kinds of dynamic processes and has direct application to nursing. All pathological and psychosocial processes can be related to the model. For example, the process of entropy or disintegration is inherent in the effects of radiation, cancer, aging, loss of adaptation, allergy, arthritis, emphysema, mental illness, and social disorganization at family and community levels. On the other hand, the process of evolution or integration explains adaptive mechanisms as immunity, specialized functioning of cells, growth, maturity of personality, mental health, and the development of hybrids in genetics and social groups. If carried to the theoretical end, the final effect of entropy is randomness to infinity or breakdown of the system. The result of evolution or integration is analogous to perfect perceptual frictionless functioning. In biological terms, the two forces of entropy and evolution are analogous to catabolism and anabolism.

The patient in his dynamic state of wellness-illness represents problems of maintenance of equilibrium of forces within his system and subsystems as well as between his system and the other systems that comprise his environment. In the state of wellness, this balance is maintained, and functioning remains close to optimum. In illness by both cause and effect, one or more of the patient's biopsychosocial systems are out of balance in respect to the forces of entropy and evolution. Usually, the process of entropy has exceeded the evolutionary force and the entropy is getting beyond the patient's ability to compensate for the strain.

The two processes, entropy and evolution, can be assessed by the nurse in the clinical setting and the assessment can be utilized as a guide for determining appropriate nursing intervention. Decisions for nursing actions are based upon the degree of presence of the opposing forces and the rate and intensity of the changes that are taking place. The rate of the reaction is at the level of kinetic theory. How fast the process is occurring varies from inertia to chaos, with speed of reactions encouraging chaotic conditions. The nurse is thus concerned with which of the processes, entropy or evolution, the patient is demonstrating as well as the rates at which the processes are proceeding. Opposing processes to varying degrees may occur simultaneously in the same patient. Through systematic observations and data collection, the patient's biopsychosocial functioning in his present situation is assessed.

When the nurse understands which of the processes are present and the rates at which the processes are proceeding, *priorities may be set* for intervention goals. Nursing intervention is aimed at counteracting the entropy with a form of evolutionary adaptation, restoring and maintaining a degree of equilibrium between the forces. The decision to be made after the goal has been determined is whether to expand, contract, or to stabilize the forces at work on the patient's subsystems as identified in the patient's state of functioning. *Expanding, contracting, or stabilizing are the only possibilities for action.* After a direction for action has been selected, the next step is to decide which nursing action can achieve the desired effect. When the appropriate nursing action has been selected, the nurse utilizes her energies and resources to supplement the patient in his state of entropy and to enhance the force of evolution so as to redirect the dynamic processes in a positive direction. When the nurse perceives that the patient is not able to cope with the increased entropy, she injects her energies to provide emotional or physical support, or both, until the patient regains enough energy to resume independent functioning. Thus, the nurse supports the patient during his dependent entropic state.

Since each of the areas identified has implications for the nursing care of every patient, assessing the processes at work permits the nurse to make rational decisions for nursing intervention designed to fit the individual patient's needs and the nursing goals that have been derived with him. The processes of entropy and evolution that are ongoing in each area of the patient's situation can be identified and explored with the intent of manipulating the situation in the patient's behalf. Nursing action, then, is based upon reason and not ritual.

Upon these hypotheses, nursing intervention can be selected and enacted. Evaluation of nursing intervention is made, then, in terms of whether the nursing action has produced the desired effect, and whether the desired effect is, in truth, the most advantageous one for the patient. Thus, the steps of the nursing process – namely, assessment, planning, intervention, and evaluation – are utilized.

The process described has its own servo-mechanism in the feedback provided through constant reassessment to correct the course of nursing action and readjust the degree of nursing intervention necessary to provide dynamic nursing care exquisitely adapted to the individual patient's situation at that time. In this model, professional nursing practice is based upon a systematic utilization of knowledge from the sciences.

To illustrate how the processes can be identified, the nurse can view the respiratory functioning of the patient in terms of entropy, or the amount of lung impairment demonstrated, and breathing exercises as an evolutionary force that aids the patient to achieve a higher level of respiratory functioning. In the cardiac system, damage to heart tissue is assessable as a degree of entropy, while rest, relaxation, and weight reduction are integrative forces that may be utilized to negate the entropy. With nutrition, the two forces may be identified in weight loss and decreased absorption, examples of entropy, as opposed to weight gain and muscle development which represent the positive integrative force. Within the nervous system, brain damage from reduced blood flow is entropic and the relearning or new learning of other functions by other areas of the brain are examples of evolutionary activity. In the psychological area, Sorensen [10] identified the dependency state of the patient during illness. This is an example

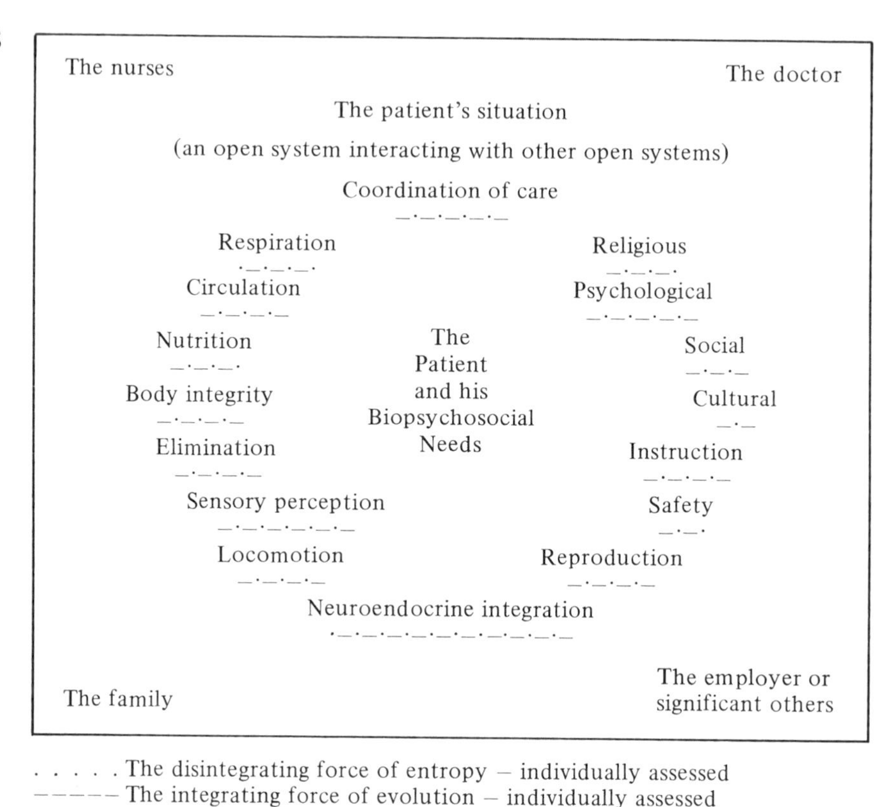

Figure 1. Concepts of general systems theory applied to nursing. (Reprinted from A. Putt, Entropy, Evolution and Equifinality in Nursing. In J. Smith (Ed.), *Five Years of Cooperation To Improve Curricula in Western Schools of Nursing.* Boulder, Colo.: Western Interstate Commission for Higher Education, 1972, p. 225.)

of a contracted entropic state. The evolutionary force in a state of dependency is the nurse, who gives of her energies to supplement the patient's reduced capacity to deal with his problems. In the social area, family disintegration is an entropic process while family solidarity is integrative. These are but a few of the many examples that could be utilized to illustrate the nature and variable degree of the processes that may be identified during systematic assessment of the patient's biopsychosocial functioning.

The concepts presented are illustrated further in Figure 1, in which the patient with his biopsychosocial needs is the center of his open system and is interacting with his individual array of other significant systems such as his family, his employer, his doctor, and his nurse or significant others. Each open system has its own semipermeable boundary and its characteristic state of equilibrium. All systems have in common an equifinality in the ultimate death of the system at some future point. The system cannot extend beyond death.

By utilizing the concepts and processes described, general systems theory can and should provide a sound guide for nursing practice and thus build a bridge from the realm of nursing theory to the reality of professional nursing practice. This is an example of "nursing's theoretical evolution" to which Newman [5] referred.

References

1. Abbey, J. C. A General Systems Approach to Nursing. In J. Smith (Ed.), *Improvement of Curricula in Schools of Nursing.* Boulder, Colo.: Western Interstate Commission for Higher Education, 1970.
2. Brillouin, L. Life, Thermodynamics, and Cybernetics. In W. Buckley (Ed.), *Modern Systems Research for the Behavioral Scientist.* Chicago: Aldine Publishing, 1968.
3. Hazzard, M. E. An overview of systems theory. *Nurs. Clin. North Am.* 6:385, 1971.
4. McKay, R. Theories, models, and systems for nursing. *Nurs. Res.* 18:393, 1969.
5. Newman, M. A. Nursing theoretical evolution. *Nurs. Outlook* 20:449, 1972.
6. Putt, A. M. Entropy, Evolution and Equifinality in Nursing. In J. Smith (Ed.), *Five Years of Cooperation to Improve Curricula in Western Schools of Nursing.* Boulder, Colo.: Western Interstate Commission for Higher Education, 1972.
7. Raymond, R. C. Communication, Entropy, and Life. In W. Buckley (Ed.), *Modern Systems Research for the Behavioral Scientist.* Chicago: Aldine Publishing, 1968.
8. Rogers, M. E. *An Introduction to the Theoretical Basis of Nursing.* Philadelphia: F. A. Davis, 1970.
9. Schrödinger, E. Order, Disorder, and Entropy. In W. Buckley (Ed.), *Modern Systems Research for the Behavioral Scientist.* Chicago: Aldine Publishing, 1968.
10. Sorensen, G. Dependency: A factor in nursing care. *Am. J. Nurs.* 66:1762, 1966.
11. von Bertalanffy, L. *General System Theory.* New York: George Braziller, 1968.

Entropy, Evolution, and Equifinality in the Nursing Process

5

Arlene M. Putt

To apply the general systems concepts to nursing practice, a guide for the systematic assessment of the patient's biopsychosocial needs is useful, because assessment of the patient's needs for nursing is the first step in providing professional nursing care. McCain [4] has declared that systematic assessment of the patient's needs is far superior to intuition in outlining the nursing care that a patient will require. While Finch [2], Geitgey [3], and McCain [4], among others [1, 6, 7], have developed guides for the assessment of patient needs, another format for a short but complete guide to patient assessment and nursing action would be useful.

A simple, but rather complete, coverage of the patient's functioning in his present situation can be achieved by assessing the processes of entropy and evolution in terms of the organ systems of the body [5]. If the patient's nursing needs can be conceived as being like spokes on a wheel, any one of which may be uppermost at a given time, but all of which are important for the support of the patient during his dysfunction, the following classification may be useful to the nurse. To assess the patient's present state of biopsychosocial functioning, the nurse interviews him and seeks information to evaluate his present state of functioning in relation to his physiological needs, psychosocial needs, and nursing concerns. The areas identified by this author for physiological assessment are respiration, circulation, nutrition, elimination, sensory perception, locomotion, neuroendocrine, reproduction, and body integrity. The psychosocial needs of individuals are divided by this author into psychological, family-oriented, social, religious, and cultural; and nursing concerns are defined as safety, instruction, and coordination of care.

While this list of areas of nursing concerns can provide a guide for a rather complete assessment of the patient in his present state of functioning, assessment is only the first step. To plan expert nursing care, the mere gathering of facts

Reprinted, with adaptations, from Entropy, Evolution, and Equifinality in Nursing. In J. Smith (Ed.), *Five Years of Cooperation to Improve Curricula in Western Schools of Nursing.* Boulder, Colo.: Western Interstate Commission for Higher Education, 1972.

 does not automatically process the facts into an appropriate plan for action. The information that has been gathered must be processed through an understanding of the forces involved. Here, the application of the theoretical framework of general systems theory is most helpful.

If one applies the concepts of entropy and evolution to the assessment process as it is enacted in nursing, one assesses the degree and rate of entropy or the amount and rate of disorganization or dysfunction that the patient displays in any of the aforementioned areas of nursing concern. Likewise, the patient can be assessed in relation to the amount and rate of integrative power or evolutionary potential that he displays in the areas of assessment. Input of energy, skill, and information from nurses, doctors, family, and significant others can also be considered evolutionary resources.

To apply these concepts to the clinical setting, basic postulates of a general systems theoretical framework can be utilized. These postulates are as follows:

1. Wellness depends upon an adequate level of biopsychosocial functioning of the individual.
2. Illness develops when the individual's biopsychosocial functioning becomes disrupted with a degenerative or disintegrative process, which can be called entropy.
3. Compensatory and coping mechanisms, which can be termed evolutionary factors, can be brought to bear upon the entropy.
4. The above process can be delineated in steps which are the nursing process leading to a plan of nursing action.

Using the above postulates as a base, the steps in developing a plan of nursing action are as follows:

1. Describe observations and findings.
2. Differentiate entropy from normal findings.
3. Describe entropy in terms of the subsystem, the degree of involvement, and the rate of change.
4. Identify compensatory and coping mechanisms in the situation – termed *evolutionary factors* – for each subsystem.
5. Weigh the balance of entropic and evolutionary factors.
6. Decide on one of the three possible goals for each entropic or evolutionary factor. The possible goals are to
   a. Enhance
   b. Stabilize
   c. Contract
7. Select nursing actions to achieve the selected goal for each system or subsystem.
8. Carry out selected nursing actions for each goal.
9. Evaluate the results of each action and reassess the remaining entropy.
10. Readjust the assessments, the goals, and the nursing actions as needed.

The University of Arizona College of Nursing Nursing Care Plan

	Entropy (−) (Problems)	Evolution (+) (Resources)	Equifinality (Goal)	Nursing Action to Achieve Goal
Physiological needs				
Respiration				
Circulation				
Nutrition				
Elimination				
Sensory perception				
Locomotion				
Neuroendocrine integration				
Reproduction				
Body integrity				
Psychosocial needs				
Psychological				
Family-oriented				
Social				
Religious				
Cultural				
Nursing concerns				
Safety				
Instruction				
Coordination of care				

Name____________________ Age________ Room________

Diagnosis____________________ Doctor________________

Figure 2. Nursing care plan

To develop a plan of nursing action, data can be recorded on the form shown as Figure 2. This brief form serves to guide the observation, recording, and processing of information into a useful plan of action.

In following the process outlined, the professional nurse evaluates the amount and rate of respiratory dysfunction and the amount and rate of the evolutionary potential or resources for assisting the respiratory functioning of the patient until the patient's respiratory entropy decreases and his evolutionary potential develops to a level of self-maintenance. Having taken the patient's respiratory functioning into account, the nurse then proceeds to assess the patient's circulatory functioning. Is the patient's circulatory entropy greater than he can cope with? Does the patient need circulatory support in terms of blood, drug therapy, or reduced activity? What is the balance that exists in the patient's circulatory functioning at this time? In like manner, the nurse evaluates each area of nursing concerns for the patient in relation to the state of balance between the degrees of entropy and the evolution present. The completed assessment provides a profile of the patient's present state of functioning.

The next steps in planning appropriate nursing care are to (1) determine priorities of concern, (2) decide on an appropriate goal, and (3) decide what nursing action is appropriate to the goal.

At this point, the third concept of the general systems theory comes into focus – the concept of equifinality as compared with multifinality. Equifinality means the sameness of the end that may be reached from varying previous states or by varying routes. Recovery from illness is one example. The patient may possibly recover with rest alone, or rest plus medication, or after other combinations of modalities. The goal – recovery – is the same, but the means to the end vary. Actually, equifinality in the form of optimum health has been in evidence in nursing for a long time. While attempts have been made in the past to espouse one correct way of providing nursing care, the reality of the situation has fostered a variety of techniques. Further examples of equifinality are health and death. One can reach either of these ends by different means. On the other hand, the means may sometimes determine the end, a concept of multifinality. In this case, the consequence of the action must be weighed in terms of the desired goal and equifinality must be distinguished from multifinality.

By utilizing an assessment guide to evaluate the forces of entropy and evolution at work in the patient's situation, the nurse must decide whether to support, to contract, or to stabilize the forces at work. These are the only possible ways to influence a system. Is the nurse going to support the patient's respiratory function with oxygen, or is she going to contract the patient's overexpanded system of hyperventilation using a rebreathing bag? Is the nurse just going to monitor the patient's circulatory functioning, or is she going to depress his heart with medication or stimulate the rate from an existing bradycardia? The equifinality desired is that of normal or near-normal functioning. Therefore, the nursing action is clearly envisioned in light of the data and the choices available to the nurse. Where normal balance exists for the patient, no further action is required by the nurse except to continue to monitor the patient's functioning periodically. Where the possibility of multifinality exists, the nurse must identify her goal and the consequences by actions in relation to that goal before selecting a choice of action.

This presentation of the patient's nursing needs can be as detailed or as brief as the situation warrants and can be summarized on the form shown as Figure 2. The more data funneled through the understanding of the processes at work, the more refined is the judgment that the nurse can make, and the more professional the nursing action can be.

References

1. Abbey, J. C. A General Systems Approach to Nursing. In J. Smith (Ed.), *Improvement of Curricula in Schools of Nursing.* Boulder, Colo.: Western Interstate Commission for Higher Education, 1970.
2. Finch, J. Systems analysis: A logical approach to professional nursing care. *Nurs. Forum* 8:177, 1969.
3. Geitgey, D. A. Self-pacing: A guide to nursing care. *Nurs. Outlook* 17:48, 1969.
4. McCain, R. F. Guide to the Systematic Assessment of the Functional Abilities of a Patient. Ann Arbor: University of Michigan School of Nursing, 1969. (Mimeographed material.)
5. Putt, A. M. Entropy, Evolution, and Equifinality in Nursing. In J. Smith (Ed.), *Five Years of Cooperation to Improve Curricula in Western Schools of Nursing.* Boulder, Colo.: Western Interstate Commission for Higher Education, 1972.
6. Ryan, B. J. Nursing care plans: A systems approach to developing criteria for planning and evaluation. *J. Nurs. Adm.* 3:(3)50, May–June, 1973.
7. Smoyak, S. A. Toward understanding nursing situations: A transaction paradigm. *Nurs. Res.* 18:405, 1969.

Assessment of Social Systems: Culture and Family 6

I. A Guide to Understanding Another Person

Arlene M. Putt

In a study of culture and stresses, Spradley and Phillips [7] explored 34 items of cultural readjustment in rank order. With a few adaptations, their work can serve as a basis for acquiring an understanding of another person's frame of reference and priorities (A Guide to Understanding Another Person, Fig. 3).

The answers to the questions raised in Spradley and Phillips' work provide considerable insight into a patient's perspectives. As shown in Figure 3, this cultural assessment can be put into a general systems framework. The concepts of entropy, evolution, and equifinality can be applied to language, pace of life and life-style. It is possible to estimate whether the components of culture, as outlined in the Guide, are in the process of disintegration or evolution. Either a static state of equilibrium or a dynamic state of rapid change is conceivable for each of the factors. The resulting assessment of culture, then, can be utilized to plan effective nursing care.

To be effective, nursing care must meet the cultural needs of the patient as well as the physiological and psychological concerns [1, 2, 3, 4, 6]. The nurse must understand the patient's milieu. This understanding can be reached by carefully identifying information about the various facets of the patient's life-style. Consideration of the cultural aspect of care is essential if the patient is to be viewed as a total human being.

The following are two examples of the use of the Guide.

The first patient is Mrs. J. B., a 37-year-old Mexican-American woman with diabetes mellitus. She was admitted to the hospital with a severe infection on her thigh. When planning appropriate care for her, the nurse will find most useful the information included in A Guide to Understanding Another Person, as summarized in Table 1 [1, 2, 3, 4, 6]. The nurse learns that the patient is fluent in both Spanish and English, that her general pace of life is leisurely, and that punctuality means within an hour or perhaps several days. Her basic diet

A Guide to Understanding Another Person

Facet	Entropy	Evolution	Equifinality
1. Language spoken			
2. General pace of life			
3. Degree of punctuality			
4. Type of food eaten			
5. General standard of living			
6. Opportunities for social contact			
7. Things found offensive			
8. Amount of ambition possessed			
9. Beliefs regarding independence of women			
10. Degree to which one engenders misunderstandings			
11. Amount of privacy desired			
12. Manner of interaction with important person			
13. Content of humor			
14. Leisure activities			
15. Personal hygiene			
16. Eating practices			
17. Amount of body contact with others			
18. Degree of formality in interpersonal relationships			
19. Ideas regarding friendships			
20. Type of transportation used			
21. Taboo subjects for conversation			
22. Expression of hospitality			
23. Treatment of children			
24. Value of material possessions			
25. Financial state			
26. Content of sadness			
27. Sense of obligation to family			
28. Race of associates			
29. Sleeping practices			
30. Significant others			
31. Type of clothes worn			
32. Religious faith			
33. Perception of work			
34. Male-female relationships			
35. Housing			
36. Employment practices			
37. Educational level			

Figure 3. A guide to understanding another person. (Adapted from J. P. Spradley and M. Phillips, Culture and Stress: A Quantitative Analysis. *Am. Anthropol.* 74:518, 1972. Reproduced by permission of the American Anthropological Association from *Am. Anthropol.* 74, 1972.)

is Mexican food, with a high ingestion of beans, tortillas, and cheese. Her standard of living is lower-class, and she and her husband live on his social security. Their home is a house trailer [2]. Opportunities for social contact are mainly through the Catholic church, the neighbors, and the extended family. Practices that Mrs. J. B. finds offensive are nudity, drug abuse, and violence. She has only a very moderate ambition to get ahead in the world and is content to do her daily tasks as a housewife. She believes that women should be subject to their husbands and she accepts her role as a homemaker and mother. Because she was raised in the Mexican culture, she tends to think along these lines and she does not always make her actions understandable to her non-Mexican-American associates. Nor does she see the need to explain her activities or to keep her word because she has given it. The amount of privacy she desires is not great, as she is accustomed to living in small quarters. Her "manner of interaction" with important persons is to remain silent; she speaks when spoken to. The content of her humor includes adventures and foibles of her pets, her children, and her relatives. For leisure, she watches daily soap operas without fail, her housework being performed during the commercials. Her personal hygiene is casual and her oral care could be improved. She is clean but informal. Eating is a social activity that consumes much of her time, as she snacks frequently, and a strong cup of black coffee is always near at hand.

Her body contact with others is limited as she usually touches only her immediate family and is touched only by them. The relationships within her large, extended family are well defined; she is polite but formal to outsiders. While she does not hesitate to use friendships to back up her activities, she does not consider that the other person involved may feel he has been "used" in the transaction. Her transportation is mainly by car, with walking limited to very short distances, such as from the house to the car. Sex and violence are taboo topics for general conversation. Her expression of hospitality is an offer of coffee and food. Children are treated with kindness and tolerance. Her material possessions are not many but they are valued highly. New furniture is one of her goals. Her financial state is precarious and limited, and the small fixed income causes her anxiety. Sadness mainly results from thinking about untoward accidents that have happened to family and friends. There is a very strong sense of obligation to her family with lesser degrees of obligation to her friends. Predominantly, her associates are Mexican-American with but few other acquaintances. She habitually retires early to a double bed with her husband; two daughters sleep in an adjoining room. Significant other persons in her life are either neighbors or relatives. Her clothing consists mainly of house dresses, pants, and tops. Catholic by faith and practice, she believes that the church is very important and its doctrines are to be followed. Work is perceived as a necessary part of life and is accepted without question. Her male-female relationships are restricted to her husband and brothers. Her home is located on a dusty street. Her employment has been restricted, as she has not worked since her marriage 16 years ago. Her husband does not want her to work. Prior to her marriage, she worked as a ticket clerk in a bus terminal. Her formal education ended in the eighth grade.

Table 1. A Guide to Understanding Another Person – Mrs. J. B., Age 37

Facet	Entropy	Evolution	Equifinality
1. Language spoken		Spanish and English	Maintain
2. General pace of life		Leisurely	Maintain
3. Degree of punctuality	Not strict		Expand
4. Type of food eaten	Mexican food		Expand
5. General standard of living	Lower class		Expand with limits
6. Opportunities for social contact		Church	Expand
7. Things found offensive		Drugs, nudity, violence	Maintain
8. Amount of ambition possessed	Low to moderate		Maintain
9. Beliefs regarding independence of women	Subject to husband – woman is homemaker		Maintain
10. Degree to which one engenders misunderstandings	Does not clarify action		Expand
11. Amount of privacy desired		Little needed	Maintain
12. Manner of interaction with important person	Is silent		Expand
13. Content of humor		Pets, friends, relatives	Maintain
14. Leisure activities	Soap operas		Expand
15. Personal hygiene	Oral hygiene deficient		Expand
16. Eating practices	Snacks	Social eating	Contract
17. Amount of body contact with others	Little		Maintain
18. Degree of formality in interpersonal relationships	Formal with nonrelatives	Informal with relatives	Maintain
19. Ideas regarding friendships	Uses friends for own purpose		Expand friends
20. Type of transportation used		Auto	Maintain
21. Taboo subjects for conversation	Sex and violence		Contract
22. Expression of hospitality		Offers coffee and food	Maintain
23. Treatment of children		Kind and tolerant	Maintain
24. Value of material possessions	High value		Contract
25. Financial state	Social security only		Maintain

Table 1 (Continued)

Facet	Entropy	Evolution	Equifinality
26. Content of sadness		Accidents to significant others	Maintain
27. Sense of obligation to family		Very strong	Maintain
28. Race of associates	Own group, Mexican-American		Expand
29. Sleeping practices		Regular pattern	Maintain
30. Significant others	Restricted to family and neighbors		Expand
31. Type of clothes worn		Casual clothes	Maintain
32. Religious faith		Strong Catholic	Maintain
33. Perception of work		Necessity	Maintain
34. Male-Female relationships	Restricted to family		Expand
35. Housing	House trailer on dirt street		Maintain
36. Employment practices	Restricted – has not worked		Maintain for present
37. Educational level	Grade school		Expand

Source: Adapted by permission from J. P. Spradley and M. Phillips, Culture and Stress: A Quantitative Analysis, *Am. Anthropol.* 74:518, 1972.

This amount of information is lengthy to gather and, in all probability, is not obtained during one interview but it is expanded with each encounter. The end result allows the nurse to plan care and instruction that are designed to fit the individual patient's situation, as illustrated in Table 2.

The second patient is Mr. J. Y., an 80-year-old blind patient with chronic congestive heart failure. He speaks English only and lives a quiet retired life on his social security money. A German-American, he is well disciplined in punctuality. He eats heavy meals of meat, potatoes, and garden vegetables with cake and pie. His general standard of living is lower middle class, and he has owned his 50-year-old, two-story brick house for many years. His opportunities for social contact are very restricted, i.e., to only his family and immediate neighbors. At the present time, he will not go outside of the house alone. He does not approve of deceit and violence. Never ambitious to get ahead, he has been content to work as a mechanic and to spend his time with his family. He believes that women really belong in the home and should obey their husbands; however, he does understand the occasional need for women to work outside the home. Basically quiet, he talks little, and thus few persons know what he is thinking. This can lead to misunderstandings. Mr. Y likes privacy. He does not like many people around him. His manner of interacting with important people is to tell small jokes. His humor concerns national figures and people he knows. His

Table 2. Nursing Care Plan – Mrs. J. B., Age 37

Area	Entropy (–) (Problems)	Evolution (+) (Resources)	Equifinality (Goal)	Nursing Action to Achieve Goal
Physiological needs				
Respiration		Normal	Maintain	Ambulate (t.i.d.)
Circulation	Atherosclerosis		Expand	Encourage movement; measure vital signs
Nutrition	Mexican-American diet		Expand	Decrease CHO intake; offer some Mexican-American food
Elimination		Normal	Maintain	Monitor function; force intake of fluids
Sensory perception		Normal	Maintain	Monitor function
Neuroendocrine	Diabetes mellitus with insulin (30 units N.P.H.)		Maintain	Give insulin; assure food availability; watch for reactions
Reproduction		Normal	Maintain	No action needed
Body integrity	Severe infection on lateral thigh		Contract infection	Administer antibiotics; observe and record; change dressings
Psychosocial needs				
Psychological	Dependent Mexican-American female		Expand	Foster her self-concept
Family-oriented		Strong family ties	Maintain	Include family in plans and teaching
Social	Restricted		Expand	Introduce her to others
Religious		Strong Catholic	Maintain	Arrange for Mass
Cultural		Mexican-American	Maintain	Offer her choices consistent with Mexican-American culture
Nursing concerns				
Safety	Infection control		Expand	Take wound precautions
Instruction	Diabetic instruction; hygiene instruction		Expand	Teach skin care; diabetic care; instruct family
Coordination of care	Surgery and medicine		Maintain	Maintain communication and coordination

Name Mrs. J. B. Age 37 Room 10

Diagnosis Diabetes mellitus with infection Doctor Smith

Source: The University of Arizona College of Nursing

leisure activities are listening to the radio or the television, or just sitting. His personal hygiene is somewhat poor at best; since he lost his sight he has had to depend on his son to shave him. His eating practice is to sit down to a full table three times a day and eat heartily. His amount of body contact with others has never been great, but since he became blind, he accepts contact from only his family. Informal with his immediate family, he is more formal with other persons. He has a few friends that have been friends for many years; he does not make new friends. Transportation modes include short walks with a family member in attendance and being driven in an automobile for greater distances. Death is a taboo subject. He withdraws from it. His expression of hospitality is to ask his visitor to sit down and talk. His treatment of children is to assert authority over them. His value of material possessions is high. While his financial state is modest, he is proud of his acquisitions and his house. Since he retired 15 years ago, he has lived on savings and social security. In addition, he has small land holdings. His blindness makes him sad, and he has never really adjusted to it. He has always felt a strong obligation to provide for his family. All his neighbors and friends are persons of German extraction, and at this time of his life he does not seek new acquaintances. His sleeping practices are regular. He retires and rises early, sleeping in a double bed with his wife of many years. Significant other persons are restricted to his family and a very few close neighbors who continue to dwindle in number. He is Protestant by faith, but he does not go to church. A hard-working man for the major part of his life, he subscribes to the Protestant work ethic. His male-female relationships are also restricted to his family and a few close neighbors. His educational level is grade school, but one of his three children is a junior college graduate. This information on Mr. Y. is summarized in Table 3.

At home he is cared for by his wife and son, with additional support from his two daughters and their families. From this it can be seen that the general systems theory format adapts itself to the planning of home care as well as to the planning of care in hospital or nursing home. A nursing care plan for Mr. Y., as he copes with his chronic congestive heart failure under home care, is summarized on page 46 in Table 4.

While a written plan is probably not needed when care is provided by a small group of people who give consistent care day after day, a written plan would be very useful to a visiting nurse or to take along to a hospital, should the need for hospital care arise [5]. Also, such a care plan would assist attendants to review whether the care they are providing is complete and adequate. If the terminology of general systems theory is too complicated for the family, the terms *things wrong, things right,* and *aims* could be substituted.

Someday perhaps such plans fusing cultural understanding and nursing care can be worked out by the nurse and the patient in the private physician's office.

Table 3. A Guide to Understanding Another Person – Mr. J. Y., Age 80

Facet	Entropy	Evolution	Equifinality
1. Language spoken		English only	Maintain
2. General pace of life	Very slow		Maintain
3. Degree of punctuality		On time	Maintain
4. Type of food eaten		German	Decrease salt
5. General standard of living		Lower middle class	Maintain
6. Opportunities for social contact	Very few		Enhance
7. Things found offensive	Deceit and violence		Maintain
8. Amount of ambition possessed	Little		Maintain
9. Beliefs regarding independence of women	Women belong at home		Maintain
10. Degree to which one engenders misunderstandings	Talks little		Enhance
11. Amount of privacy desired	Seeks seclusion		Enhance
12. Manner of interaction with important person	Tells small jokes		Maintain
13. Content of humor		People-oriented	Maintain
14. Leisure activities	Sitting and listening		Enlarge
15. Personal hygiene	Cannot shave self		Encourage
16. Eating practices		3 meals per day	Maintain
17. Amount of body contact with others	Little		Encourage
18. Degree of formality in interpersonal relationships	Formal outside family		Maintain
19. Ideas regarding friendships	Few old friends		Enhance
20. Type of transportation used		Auto and walking	Encourage discussion
21. Taboo subjects for conversation	Death		Encourage
22. Expression of hospitality		Sit and talk	Encourage
23. Treatment of children	Asserts authority		Maintain
24. Value of material possessions		High	Maintain
25. Financial state		Modest	Maintain
26. Content of sadness	Blindness		Encourage

Table 3 (Continued)

Facet	Entropy	Evolution	Equifinality
27. Sense of obligation to family		Strong	Maintain
28. Race of associates		German-American	Maintain
29. Sleeping practices	Regular		Maintain
30. Significant others	Few		Encourage
31. Type of clothes worn		Work clothes	Maintain
32. Religious faith		Protestant	Encourage
33. Male-female relationships		Male dominance	Maintain
34. Housing		Owns large house	Maintain
35. Employment practices	Retired and blind		Status quo
36. Educational level	Grade school		Status quo

Source: Adapted by permission from J. P. Spradley and M. Phillips, Culture and Stress: A Quantitative Analysis, *Am. Anthropol.* 74:518, 1972

References

1. Branch, M., and Paxon, P. *Providing Safe Nursing Care for Ethnic People of Color.* New York: Appleton-Century-Croft, 1976.
2. Bullough, B., and Bullough, V. L. *Poverty, Ethnic Identity, and Health Care.* New York: Appleton-Century-Croft, 1972.
3. Clark, M. *Health in the Mexican-American Culture* (2d ed.). Berkeley, Calif.: University of California Press, 1970.
4. Kosa, J., Antonovsky, A., and Zola, I. (Eds.), *Poverty and Health, A Sociological Analysis.* Cambridge: Harvard University Press, 1969.
5. Roberts, S. L. *Behavioral Concepts and the Critically Ill Patient.* Englewood Cliffs, N.J.: Prentice-Hall, 1976.
6. Spicer, E. Southwestern Healing Traditions in the 1970s: An Introduction. In E. Spicer (Ed.), *Ethnic Medicine in the Southwest.* Tucson: The University of Arizona Press, 1977.
7. Spradley, J. P., and Phillips, M. Culture and stress: A quantitative analysis. *Am. Anthropol.* 74:518, 1972.

Table 4. Nursing Care Plan – Mr. J. Y., Age 80

Area	Entropy (–) (Problems)	Evolution (+) (Resources)	Equifinality (Goal)	Nursing Action to Achieve Goal
Physiological needs				
Respiration	Chews tobacco	Does not smoke	Maintain	Discourage tobacco
Circulation	Chronic congestive heart failure	On digitoxin 0.1 mg p.o. q.d.	Maintain	Encourage slow pace
Nutrition	Overweight	Eats regular meals	Contract	Decrease salt and heavy food
Elimination	Constipated, enlarged prostate	Function still adequate	Maintain	Encourage fluids and walking; observe output
Sensory perception	Blind	Good hearing	Maintain	Encourage usual activities
Locomotion	Sedentary	No arthritis	Encourage	Encourage to walk to limits
Neuroendocrine	Normal		Maintain	No action
Reproduction	80 years old		Maintain	No action
Body integrity	Cannot see skin		Maintain	Have family inspect regularly
Psychosocial needs				
Psychological	Reduced self-esteem	Achieved his goals of family rearing	Encourage	Point out positive aspects
Family-oriented	Small family	Close-knit	Maintain	No action
Social	Recluse		Encourage	Arrange new contacts
Religious	Nonpracticing			No action
Cultural		Single culture (German-American)	Maintain	No action
Nursing concerns				
Safety	Blindness, age		Maintain	Remove obstacles
Instruction	Age, blindness		Encourage	Explain repeatedly; instruct family
Coordination of care	Health, age, blindness	Family care	Maintain	No action

Name Mr. J. Y. Age 80 Room 5A

Diagnosis Blindness, congestive heart failure Doctor Jones

Source: The University of Arizona College of Nursing

II. The Normal Growing Family

Arlene M. Putt

While many of the illustrations given have been derived from the area of medical-surgical nursing, the general systems theory approach is equally applicable to situations in pediatrics, obstetrics, psychiatry, and family and community nursing. An illustration of this point is an application of general systems theory to the nursing plans for a young family with a 4-year-old child and a second child on the way [1, 2].

The K.'s are in their early thirties and have been married for 10 years; they have a 4-year-old daughter. Mrs. K. is a high school teacher and is now 5 months pregnant with the second child. Mr. K. is a business man who spends long hours at the office. The family situation can be approached from a nursing plan that encompasses the entire family as a total unit or from the view that the family is composed of three individuals who are interrelated. To clarify the different approaches, a nursing plan will be worked out both ways so that the reader can compare, contrast, and then choose which approach better meets his own applications.

First, let us add more information on the family. The K.'s live in a neat, middle-class neighborhood of individual homes on one-third of an acre in the residential section of a southwestern metropolitan area. They have lived at this address for the past 2½ years, after having bought the house at the urging of friends who were also friends of the neighbors next door. Neither of the K.'s parents live nearby; both sets of parents live across the country. The only nearby relative is a sister of Mrs. K., who lives about 100 miles away.

Mr. and Mrs. K. are young, basically healthy adults of English descent. Mr. K. does not appear to have any health problems. Mrs. K. has varicosities and allergies to various pollens.

Mr. K. is established in his business as a real estate salesman. In his spare time he plays with his daughter or works at home improvement projects, creates metal sculpture, does silversmithing, and engages in target-shooting.

Mrs. K. works part time as a high school teacher, while the 4-year-old daughter is cared for by a nearby babysitter. In addition, Mrs. K. has begun to teach one night class for the local community college. Mrs. K.'s first pregnancy ended in 6 hours of labor with postdelivery hemorrhage. At the present time Mrs. K. is finding that the long hours of being on her feet, along with her pregnancy, are causing fatigue and aching legs. To reduce her fatigue, Mrs. K. wears support hose during her work and tries to get adequate rest and good nutrition. Mrs. K. does her housework and cares for her child after she comes home but she is avoiding heavy lifting. She has no assistance with her housework other than when her husband occasionally takes over a household chore while she prepares for classes and grades papers. Mrs. K. is preparing her child for the arrival of the new baby by discussing the changes in her body as they occur. Recently, Mrs. K. had a bout of headaches which subsided after she reduced her sodium intake as suggested by the school nurse.

The child, Susan, was born after a moderate labor during which her mother had tranquilizers but no other sedatives. Susan is a bright, active 4-year-old who is beginning to read and is starting to play more aggressively as she goes through a rapid spurt of growth.

While Susan plays with other children at the babysitter's, a big need at this time is a close playmate. A little girl friend lives down the street, but the children are still too young to visit back and forth without adult supervision. When Susan gets lonely she invents a sister and tells stories of what she and her sister do. Susan spends much of her time with adults and with her dog. At the present time, Susan is at the stage of giving the dog many and repeated directions. The dog, a German shepherd, grows weary of this barrage of orders and seeks relief by going to the adults and ignoring the child's commands. Because of the time she spends with adults, Susan regularly participates in adult activities and converses freely in excellent grammar. Susan's other playmate is her 7-year-old cousin, who visits about once or twice a month. When her parents are busy, Susan spends some of her time with the woman next door, helping her in the garden. Susan watches *Sesame Street* regularly and receives *Highlights for Children* magazine. As Susan grows older, she is expected to assume some responsibilities for household chores. She has learned to make her bed and to pick up her toys. She is learning to help with other activities in preparation for the new baby.

A new outlet for Susan is Sunday school. She has started to attend a Protestant Sunday school and finds this a pleasant experience in which she is making new friends. Susan's only health problem is a tendency to have recurrent respiratory infections; however, these have been fewer this past year since she has had a spurt of rapid growth and has become more physically active in riding her tricycle, swimming, and working out on her swing set.

In utilizing a care plan for the entire family, the areas usually considered separately for each individual might be considered in toto for the entire group. For instance, all the physical problems of all the family members are included together, as are all the psychosocial considerations and their interrelatedness, and finally the nursing concerns, as illustrated in Table 5.

The other approach that can be utilized is to consider each area separately for each member of the family. This is the approach utilized in Table 6, page 50. In utilizing this approach, the mother, the father, and the child are assessed individually and the reader interrelates the information. The reader may decide which of the two approaches to family care plans is better suited to his own frame of reference.

References

1. Blair, C., and Salerno, E. *The Expanding Family: Childbearing.* Boston: Little, Brown, 1976.
2. Clark, A., and Affonso, D. *Childbearing: A Nursing Perspective.* Philadelphia: F. A. Davis, 1976.

Table 5. Nursing Care Plan for K. Family Considered In Toto

Area	Entropy (–) (Problems)	Evolution (+) (Resources)	Equifinality (Goal)	Nursing Action to Achieve Goal
Physiological needs	Mother has varicosities and allergies to pollen 4 mo. of pregnancy to go Recent bout of headaches 4-yr.-old Susan has history of recurrent respiratory infections	Healthy young parents Mother 5 mo. pregnant Nonsmoker Second child Pregnancy uncomplicated No drug intake Child basically healthy	Maintain and encourage family development	Encourage mother to wear support hose Urge mother to get adequate rest and nutrition Check child's nutrition and development Urge father to quit smoking School R.N. urged mother to cut sodium intake – she did and headaches disappeared Encourage husband to aid wife in household chores Encourage child to develop responsibility for small chores Praise her attempts
All other systems normal	Husband smokes 1½ packs a day	Father major wage earner; supportive of family members		
Psychosocial needs	Child has few playmates	Child – 4-yr.-old bright, preschooler Socializes with adults	Encourage growth – physical development	Foster reading, active play Plan for sibling Prepare child for sibling Encourage socialization with other children
Cultural		White American – middle class		
Religion		Protestant – mother and child irregular in attendance		
Nursing concerns Instruction		Both parents college graduates Child very bright	Encourage	Teach prenatal care and planning Plan with family as unit for new baby
Safety		Child understands poisons and follows directions		Explain safety needs of new baby to 4-yr.-old child
Coordination of care		Mother takes no medication, nonsmoker, under care of OBS/M.D. and school R.N.		

Table 6. Nursing Care Plan for K. Family Viewed as Individuals

Area	Entropy (–) (Problems)	Evolution (+) (Resources)	Equifinality (Goal)	Nursing Action to Achieve Goal
Mother				
Physiological needs				
Respiration	Allergies to pollen		Avoid pollen	Encourage to avoid pollen
Circulation	Varicosities		Contract	Encourage to wear support hose
Reproductive	4 months to go	5 mo. pregnant	Maintain normal pregnancy	Maintain adequate diet Avoid excess salt Avoid drugs and toxins
Other systems		Normal	Maintain	Maintain health practices
Psychosocial needs				
Psychological		Happy with pregnancy	Support self identity	
Social		Happy with role of wife and mother	Maintain family role	Encourage family activities
Cultural		White American – middle class	Maintain culture	Encourage community activity
Religion		Goes to church occasionally; Protestant	Maintain religion	Encourage religious participation
Nursing concerns				
Instruction			Encourage further learning	Teach nutrition and exercise
Safety			Reinforce safety practices	Avoid toxins
Coordination of care				Coordinate assistance from RN in school and OBS
Father				
Physiological needs				
Respiration	Smokes 1–1½ packs a day	No respiratory problems to date	Enhance health	Talk with father re nonsmoking
Other systems		Normal	Maintain	Support health habits

Psychosocial needs				
Psychological		Happy with role of father, wage earner	Support self-identity	Support masculine role
Social		Easy going; successful man	Maintain social contacts	Encourage his assistance of wife with her chores
Cultural		White American businessman	Maintain culture	
Religion	Nonparticipating			
Child				
Physiological needs				
Respiration	Frequent respiratory infections	Active in exercises	Enhance exercises	Encourage active play Protect child from respiratory infections
Nutrition		Rapid growth period	Foster growth	Encourage nutritional snacks
Psychosocial needs				
Development	Few playmates	Rapid development of self and social being Sunday school contacts Plays with her dog and neighbor		Spend time with child in play activities Teach child re new baby
Nursing concerns				
Instructions and safety				Teach child safety, hazards to avoid

III. The Pathological Family

Mary Ellen Hazzard

The application of general systems theory to family therapy may produce effective outcomes with pathological families. It is a framework that can be used by the therapist to catalyze the family into changing its pathological interaction, thereby allowing the symptomatic member to give up destructive behavior.

Hall [3] defines a system as a set of units with common properties where the state of one unit is dependent upon the state of the other units. A family is a group of individuals banded together by the common interests of its members. The welfare of one family member is likely to depend upon the welfare of the other members. Man's family can, therefore, be thought of and studied as a system.

The degree of openness of a system is gauged by the amount of energy exchange between the system and its surroundings. Generally, healthy family systems are open systems with members freely exchanging materials and information with their environment. In pathological families, energy exchange is decreased and the open-family system becomes a closed system. When there is decreased interaction within a family system and between the system and its surroundings, the family becomes dysfunctional. A disrupted family system can, with time and assistance, become more organized and open. When a disorganized family is assisted toward a change in its behavior, the members discover that change is possible. Though the process is painful, with appropriate support and confrontation by the therapist, a family system can become healthier, and its members more effective in meeting their needs. The family's energies, rather than going off on a tangent, are then utilized to support the existing system of family relationships.

When general systems theory is used as the framework for helping disrupted families, the therapeutic process is directed to the family system as a whole without attention to the individuals involved at the time [1]. Change within the system is viewed as the desirable goal, although for the pathological family, it may only be a goal of maintenance of the status quo. Responsibility for change in the relationship system lies within the family, the therapist acting only as a catalyst for change rather than a change agent.

Family relationship therapy helps individual family members disengage themselves from the disorganized family system. This approach to family emotional illness utilizes the concept of wholeness in that a change in one part of the system (family interaction) is followed by a compensatory change in other parts of the system, the symptomatic members [2].

The task of the therapist who uses general systems theory in family relationship therapy is to describe the family relationship system, identify its processes of entropy and evolution, assist the family members to examine the mechanisms as they are operating, and to catalyze behavior changes of family members who strive to reach a better mode of interaction.

In order to understand how a pathological family system operates, it is first necessary to gather data on members of the immediate and extended families. A family's history should span at least three generations. Historical information to be collected includes data on each family member such as birth date, death, major illness or hospitalization, marriage and divorce, change in occupational or financial status, and individual family feuds and alliances. Once the information has been obtained, a family history diagram can be constructed by recording the important dates, years, and critical family happenings on a three-generation chart of the family tree. Intense family relationships, such as between a mother and son, can be plotted by drawing connecting dotted lines between the two family members. The resulting family diagram is then used by the therapist to describe the family's operational system. The therapist, along with the family, can use the chart to identify the dynamic processes in operation within the pathological relationship system (Fig. 4).

Family assessment and intervention can be demonstrated by the following discussion of a clinical example of a pathological family.

Initial contact with the M. family occurred 2 weeks after Jeanne M., aged 43, was discharged from the State Mental Hospital. The family was referred by the hospital social worker to the County Health Department's nurse therapist for psychiatric counseling and family therapy.

On visiting the home, the therapist found the M. family living in a row house situated in a low-to-medium-priced neighborhood on the outskirts of the city. On the outside, the house looked like all the other houses on the street except that it was more in need of paint and repair – it was shabby in comparison to the other houses in the block.

Bob, aged 42, opened the door. He was stocky, dark haired, and very nervous. Jeanne M. and four of the five M. children were gathered together in the dark and run-down living room. Elizabeth, aged 20, was not there because she was married and had a family and home of her own outside of the nuclear family.

The M. family appeared uncomfortable about the upcoming interview. Bob took a seat by himself, on the other side of the room, while Jeanne and the three boys sat close together on the couch. Chuck, aged 18, sat next to his mother, slouched down in his seat; he looked alternately at Bob, at Jeanne, and at the therapist. He was long-haired, barefooted, and dressed in dirty jeans. His brothers, Bill and Danny, aged 17 and 14, with their short hair and clean clothes, contrasted sharply with Chuck's unconventional appearance. Martha, who was 12 years old, wanted to go outside and play. Both she and Danny appeared disinterested and bored by the transactions going on among the other members of the family.

Bob acted friendly toward the therapist, but he seemed to have already made up his mind about the outcome of the home visit. His "what's the use" attitude was not shared by Jeanne, who wore a faded housedress, worn slippers, and stockings that bagged down around her ankles. She desperately wanted the family's problems solved, but not necessarily by the family itself! Her eagerness and need for the family to be helped caused her to look breathless and anxious

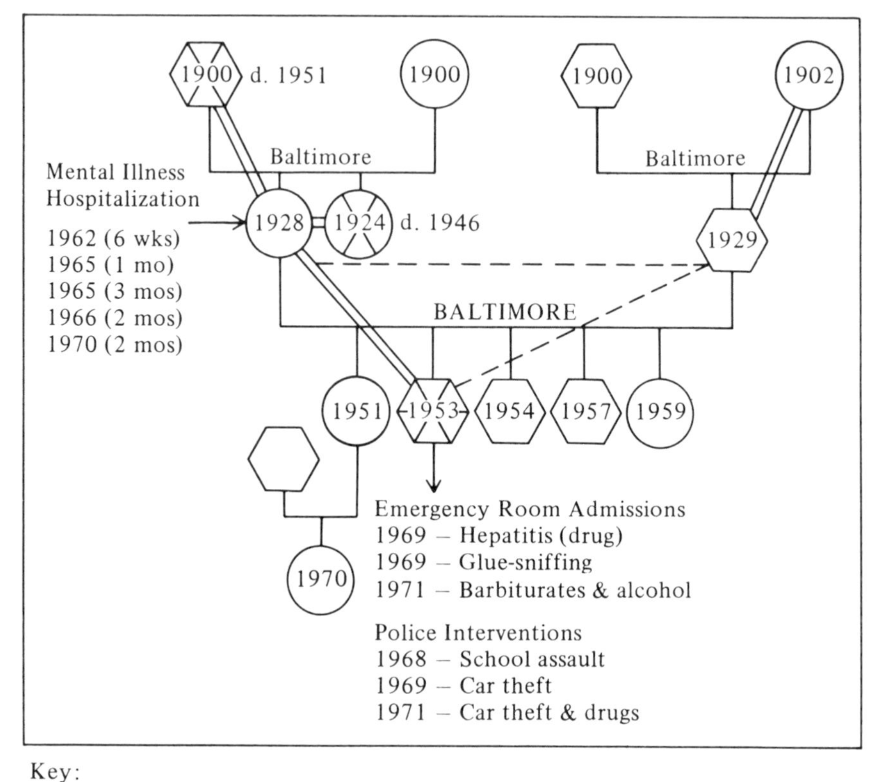

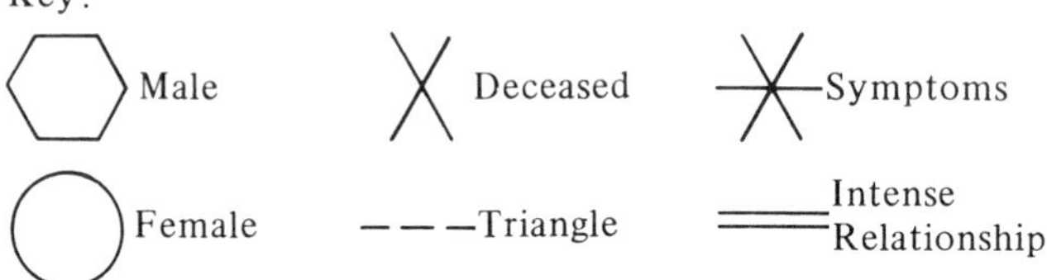

Figure 4. Family history diagram – operational system: immediate and extended fami

throughout the interview. She fidgeted in her seat, picked at her fingernails, and twisted her hair – she actually seemed to be on the verge of panic.

During the history-taking, the family members interacted freely with the therapist; however, they did not interact openly or freely with each other.

Jeanne, the family historian, frequently interrupted or corrected the stories being told by the other family members. Chuck shifted in his seat and acted sullen by refusing to volunteer information about himself or about the family. When asked a direct question, he answered in a bored, monotonous tone of voice; however, he was not unaffected by the family's interactions, for he smirked and seemed to enjoy the scene.

In retaliation to both Jeanne and Chuck, Bob remained silent and withdrawn during most of the family interview.

Chuck had quit school in his junior year of high school. He was labeled a problem student because he had difficulty getting along with his teachers and with his peers. He was not self-motivated and he did not seem interested in learning. His acting-out behavior in school included poor school attendance and unprovoked attacks on other students. In the last two years, he had been arrested three times – once for assaulting another student, once for stealing a car, and once for the possession and use of drugs. He is now on probation to both the city and county courts and assigned to the custody of his parents. This was Chuck's third offense, and according to Bob, he should have been in jail. Chuck had been treated in the hospital emergency room three times during the past 3 years – the first admission was for drug-related hepatitis, another was for glue-sniffing, while the last one was for acute barbiturate and alcohol overdose. As a result of these admissions, Chuck was ordered in for counseling as an outpatient at the mental health center. To date, he has not responded to either the psychiatric therapy or to the drug rehabilitation program. Despite his being on probation, Chuck continues his former life-style of staying out late, sometimes not coming home for several days, taking drugs along with his friends, and stealing cars for joyriding around the city. Unable to control Chuck, Bob and Jeanne protect him by keeping silent when the probation officer questions Chuck about his activities. Their conspiracy of silence encourages Chuck to continue his delinquent behavior.

Conflict between the spouses started shortly after their marriage 20 years ago. It increased after the birth of their first child. Bob's mother disliked Jeanne, and she developed the habit of criticizing her in front of Bob. She wanted Jeanne to take care of the baby her way, since it was her only grandchild. Jeanne resented the meddling and asked Bob to tell his mother not to interfere. Instead, Bob, who was very close to his mother, took her side against Jeanne. This made Jeanne angry and in a fit of rage, she ordered Bob's mother out of the house. Jeanne's feud with her mother-in-law lasted over a year and ended only after Bob promised to take her side against his mother.

The birth of each child increased the couple's marital problems – the theme of the conflict was always their children. Bob wanted obedience and respect – especially from Chuck. Since he was inclined to overcontrol and manipulate, Bob was never able to establish his sought-after father-son relationship with Chuck. They sparred continually to see which one of them could gain control over the family.

The home is a battleground for the two men, as they openly clash over one issue after another. Bob, hoping to change Chuck's behavior, criticizes and belittles him in front of his friends. Chuck, in turn, gets back at his father by staying out later, letting his hair grow longer, getting drunker, and acting lazier. He learned early how to use his so-called shortcomings as devices to needle his father.

Chuck's greatest shortcoming, according to Bob, is not finishing high school, and even though Chuck is enrolled in an adult vocational program learning how to repair cars, Bob still sees him as a failure. Education is very important to

Bob, for his long-range goal was to obtain a college degree. To this end, he has worked as a civil engineer in a steel plant during the day and in the evening attends night school. He has been pursuing his goal for the last 5 years, but considering what is now occurring in the family, he no longer expects to reach his objective.

Bob is obsessed with the idea of education while Jeanne is possessed with the urge to mother others. She has an abnormal need to control, to think, to feel, and to live for her children. She is an emotional overfunctioner and her behavior within the family has caused the children to react negatively toward her. When rejected by them, she becomes angry, unhappy, and aggressively mute. In child-rearing, she will not tolerate Bob's interference. She always makes excuses for the children, and takes their side against Bob in family arguments. Since Jeanne does not see Bob as much of a man, she treats him with belligerence and contempt.

Jeanne's father died when she was 23 years old. His death, along with the death of her sister 5 years earlier, left a great void in her life. While Jeanne was growing up, she liked to pretend that she was taking care of her father. After graduation from high school, her motherly drives and the desire to take care of people helped her make the decision to become a nurse. She married Bob 2 months after graduating from nurses' training. She wanted to take care of him and it was a great disappointment to her when Bob continued to rely on his mother for advice and emotional support.

Jeanne never worked full time and she never considered herself a practicing nurse. Her last job was 8 years ago, when she worked as a city jail nurse. It was during this time that she sought psychiatric treatment. She complained of insomnia, hallucinations, delusions, and paranoid thoughts. She blamed her symptoms on the worry and stress created by her job at the jail and by her problems at home with Bob and the children. Her symptoms grew worse, and later that year she was hospitalized for mental illness. At State Hospital, where she stayed for 6 weeks, she was diagnosed as a chronic schizophrenic.

Jeanne was hospitalized 5 times over the next 8 years. The length of each hospital admission varied from 1 to 2 months, with her longest symptom-free period being 3 years. While Jeanne was away from home, her mother took over the household. Jeanne resented her mother's intrusion into her family so much that after her last hospitalization she ordered her mother out of the house. They have not seen each other since and Jeanne refuses to correspond with her mother, who has since moved to Canada. Jeanne insists that she is able to care for her family; however, her short periods of remission belie her ability to cope with the family's overwhelming tension and discord.

The M. family is caught up in the entropy of their system – albeit the members' degree of involvement and their emotional need structure determine their ability to cope with the family's disorganized behavior patterns. The second son, Bill, tries to keep a low profile, but when forced to choose sides, he stands with Chuck and his mother. Bob seems not to have the same intense negative feelings toward Bill that he has toward Chuck. Bill, like Chuck, is learning how to be an automobile mechanic, but he also appears to be more his own man. This was evidenced by his electing to leave the family meeting after the first hour.

As for Martha and Danny, they too, are outside the family triad – since

Chuck has already been labeled by the family as its symptomatic member, they try to remain on the sidelines and uninvolved in the emotional triangle. Both Martha and Danny have emotional and school problems, and 6 months ago, the school counselor referred them to the school psychologist for diagnosis and treatment. They are currently seeing a child psychologist at the nearby mental health clinic.

The stage was set for family therapy at the end of the first session when the therapist explained to the family the meaning of family dynamics and its role in family relationship therapy. Based on the family's interaction pattern, the therapist elected to work with Jeanne, Bob, and Chuck. These three family members are more emotionally fused than the other members of the family, and, hence, they make up the family's emotional triangle. It was explained to them that the objective of relationship therapy was to get the partners to modify their patterns of interaction. Since the members' anxiety level was high and their ego fusion not too severe, modification of their system was possible. Modification of the system effects change by allowing the partners to make a project out of themselves, thus breaking up the triangle and defocusing the symptomatic member who, in the M. family, is Chuck.

Discussion

Bowen's Differentiation of Self Scale [2] was used to conceptualize emotional functioning within the M. family. Theoretically, a profile of complete differentiation of self is equivalent to complete emotional maturity and has an assigned value of 100 on a scale ranging from 0 to 100. The M. family, according to their history, falls into the lowest quarter of the scale (0 to 25). Bowen considers individuals in this scale range as more emotionally fused and less differentiated than those persons in the higher scale categories. He goes on to describe the "fused" as living in a "feeling" world, that is, if they are not too miserable to feel! Their life's energies are directed at maintaining the system – into loving and being loved, or reacting against not being loved. At best, there is a dearth of energy left in their system to attempt a more mature level of functioning. Persons at this level are incapable of using the differentiated "I" in their relationships with others. Their use of "I" is confined to what they want or what they feel, and their survival depends upon the development of emotional attachments similar to their parental ego mass. From these dependent attachments, they manage to borrow enough ego strength to function [2].

The M. family is a good example of this level of emotional functioning. Decision-making is always a major crisis; and decisions once made are usually ineffectively carried out. When things become difficult and family discord increases, Jeanne retreats into her world of mental illness, while Bob, rejecting the "I" stand in family functioning, throws up his hands and withdraws. The family's energies are invested in obtaining immediate symptomatic relief and comfort. They will accept any services that will assist them in maintaining themselves at their present level of functioning.

According to Bowen [2], spouses use three major mechanisms to control the intensity of ego fusion, (1) *marital conflict,* (2) *dysfunction of one spouse,* and (3) *transmission of problems to one or more children.* All three mechanisms are being used by the M. family. *Marital conflict* is evidenced by the relationship between the spouses. As for child-rearing, Jeanne stands at one end of a continuum with Bob at the other – they hold emotionally charged, intense, and opposite viewpoints about the proper upbringing and treatment of children. This unresolved difference of opinions is a symptom of their immature marriage.

Bob's behavior within the family is an example of the *dysfunction of one spouse.* He exudes inadequacy. He habitually withdraws from problems, and in doing so reaches a state of "no self." Jeanne's emotional excesses result in her seeking to dominate the household by constant doing and controlling – she takes responsibility for finding jobs for the boys, making doctors' appointments, school schedules, and so on. Her overfunctioning is probably a carry-over from the family origin where, as the oldest sister, she assumed the role of taking care of others [5].

The phenomenon of "overadequate–inadequate reciprocity" is used to maintain emotional balance between the spouses. In essence, this means that if one spouse assumes family leadership and direction, the other spouse may withdraw toward a state of passivity. Each complains of being dominated by the other.

The third mechanism, *transmission of problems to the siblings,* shows up in the triad between Jeanne, Bob, and Chuck. The emotional bond among the three is extremely fused – they are as one. Chuck takes full advantage of the situation by exploiting both parents through manipulative behavior. He admittedly enjoys his position in the family system, since he is always in focus!

Therapeutic Intervention

Therapeutic interventions were designed to accomplish tasks in relation to the three major mechanisms previously discussed:

1. Resolve marital conflicts
2. Motivate both spouses to function
3. Eliminate sibling symptoms

Foremost of these is the marital conflict [4]. Most therapy sessions were structured to deal with the marital dyad. It was thought that the spouse dysfunction and acting-out of the children were signs of parental distress. Therefore, if the marital conflicts could be resolved, both other symptoms would dissipate. Marital therapy, then, focused on the major area of conflict – power struggles over the children's upbringing. First, a detailed history of each partner was taken to help the spouses see how their past family relationship might be contributing to their current conflicts. The family diagram shows the extended and nuclear families of both spouses and their operant emotional relationship systems (Fig. 4).

Then, expectations for children's behavior were explored. Both Bob and

Jeanne were found to be lacking in information about normal growth and development. Many of their expectations were unrealistic and needed to be examined.

Findings indicated that therapy should center upon ventilation of the couple's feelings, development of realistic expectations on their part for their children and for each other, and avoidance of laying blame. Since most of Bob's and Jeanne's time was spent in blaming each other for their problems, the therapist made a contract with both Bob and Jeanne for each to accept responsibility for his own behavior and feelings. They were helped to develop *together* a new set of rules for their children, and they contracted with the therapist to enforce them jointly.

Gradually, as the parents learned to work together and to be consistent with their children, the children, particularly Chuck, stopped their acting-out behavior. This validated the hypothesis that their behavior was a symptom of marital conflict. Once Bob and Jeanne were able to develop and accept their own individual identities, they were then able to extend their respect for each of their children as individuals. Chuck no longer needed to manipulate his parents because they gave him the attention he needed. Change in one part of a system produces change in the whole.

Jeanne's and Bob's sexual problems were also a symptom of their immature marriage. Once they learned to communicate on a different level, they were able to ease their sexual tension. Exercises in learning their own sexual needs, then communicating those needs to each other, alleviated this symptom.

When the therapist had terminated treatment of the M. family, most of the goals of the therapy had been met; but the family made a request to continue, so they were referred to the mental health clinic for additional family relationship therapy.

Nursing Care Plan

One alternative to planning therapy for the M. family is to use a systems theory care plan. The M. family care plan (Table 7, p. 60) is included to serve as an example of how the systems approach can be used to develop therapeutic interventions into a care plan for a pathological family.

References

1. Bowen, M. Intrafamily Dynamics in Emotional Illness. In A. D'Agostino (Ed.), *Family, Church, and Community*. New York: P. J. Kennedy and Sons, 1965.
2. Bowen, M. The use of family theory in clinical practice. *Compr. Psychiatry* 7:3, 1966, pp. 346, 347, 351, 357, 373.
3. Hall, A. D., and Fagen, R. E. Definition of Systems. In W. Buckley (Ed.), *Modern Systems Research for the Behavioral Scientist*. Chicago: Aldine Publishing, 1968, pp. 81–86.
4. Hazzard, M. E., and Scheuerman, M. Family systems therapy: New way to help families in trouble. *Nursing 76* 6(7):22–23, 1976.
5. Toman, W. *Family Constellation*. New York: Springer Publishing, 1969, pp. 114–121, 129, 145–149.

Table 7. Nursing Care Plan – The M. Family

Areas	Entropy (–) (Problems)	Evolution (+) (Resources)	Equifinality (Goal)	Nursing Action to Achieve Goal
Physiological needs				
Body's systems		Normal	Maintain	
Psychosocial-cultural needs				
Marital conflict	Relationship between spouses		Contract by: Identifying family relationships that might contribute to current conflict	Deal with marital dyad Obtain family history
	Spouses' power struggles over children's upbringing		Contract by: Developing realistic expectations of children	Provide information on growth and development
			Developing together new set of rules for children	
			Jointly enforcing new set of rules	Support decisions
	Spouses' sexual relationship		Expand by: Meeting each other's needs	Provide sex counseling
	Family finances		Maintain to expand with limits	Refer to social agencies
Dysfunction of one spouse	Inadequacy: Bob's withdrawing from family problems		Contract by: Ventilating feelings	Help identify blame-laying behavior Support decisions
	Jeanne's emotional overfunctioning: overcontrol of family members		Accepting responsibility for own behavior and feelings Feeling less responsible for others	Help identify blame-laying behavior Encourage reality-testing Discourage over-protective behavior

	Bob's depression		Contract by: Improving self-image	Establish rapport Build a trust relationship Encourage ventilation of feelings
	Low self-esteem		Relating better to others Mobilizing and using own resources Improving ability to deal with stress	Point out family's assets Manipulate environment Help family communicate more effectively
	Jeanne's chronic mental illness: thought disorder	Under care of therapist	Maintain by: Correctly interpreting internal and external stimuli	Respond to feelings Capitalize on ego assets Encourage reality thinking Stress responsibility for own behavior
			Relating to others	Support decision-making via encouragement Communicate openly and clearly Give honest feedback on interpretation of data
Sibling's symptoms	Chuck's acting-out behavior: Manipulation Drug-abuse		Contract by: Accepting responsibility for own decisions and behaviors Improving judgment and decision-making ability Improving interpersonal relationships	Help parents to develop realistic expectations of children by: Setting limits Being consistent and firm Creating atmosphere for expression of needs in an honest and open manner Willingness to negotiate
		Mental health counseling	Maintain by: Continued counseling	Identify manipulative behaviors
Educational		Men trying to improve education	Maintain and expand	Support family's objectives
Social	No social interaction		Expand	Encourage family to increase social activities

A Nursing Care Plan Using a General Systems Framework 7

Arlene M. Putt

To illustrate the concepts of general systems theory in nursing practice, an example has been extracted from clinical nursing. Miss J., a 23-year-old woman with cerebral palsy, was hospitalized for a trial on the drug levodopa (L-dopa). Because of the new surroundings and the patient's lack of fine motor control, her safety was a high priority. The data for the assessment of this patient were gathered while the author was assisting her with her tub bath; the time required to write up the assessment was less than 15 minutes. In this short time, the data were recorded, the forces identified, the priorities evaluated, and appropriate nursing actions delineated. For many patients, however, more time might be required for the completion of the plan. Moreover, for this patient it may be necessary to add information as it becomes available in the future.

Physiological Needs

The assessment of Miss J.'s nursing needs was as follows: in her *respiratory* functioning, Miss J. displayed entropy in the form of athetoid respiration and a weak cough. Her respiratory entropy was offset by an evolutionary process of continuous movement. The goal regarding her respiratory functioning was to maintain her active state and to strengthen her cough. Thus, the nursing action in relation to her respiratory functioning was to encourage deep breathing and coughing. Miss J.'s circulation was normal, and the goal was simply to maintain this circulatory function. Reassessment was made by the nursing action of monitoring the vital signs periodically. In relation to *nutrition,* Miss J.'s intake and digestion were normal, but entropy was apparent in her continuous muscular movement, which expended great amounts of energy. The nutritional goal for this patient was to maintain her food intake at a high level, and the nursing action was to encourage the intake of a high-caloric diet to compensate for her continuous activity. Miss J. had no problems with elimination by either bowel or bladder, so the goal was to maintain this normal functioning; excretion was monitored as needed.

While most of Miss J.'s *sensory perception* was normal, she had a nerve deafness for which she compensated with a hearing aid. The nursing goal was to maintain Miss J.'s hearing at its present level, to check and safeguard her hearing aid, and to speak slowly in front of her.

In *locomotion,* Miss J. had pronounced entropy in the form of continuous gross movements and contracted heel tendons. To compensate, the patient was on a routine of exercises for 20 minutes 4 times a day as prescribed by her physician and her physical therapist. The goal was to maintain her level of functioning through the regular use of the exercises. The nurse had only to provide space and safety while Miss J. did her exercises.

In *neuroendocrine functioning,* Miss J. had great entropy in the form of severe cerebral palsy with continuous athetoid movement. Her neurological functioning was compensated for by very high intelligence. Her endocrine functioning appeared normal. As an attempt at evolution, the drug levodopa was being initiated with the hope that increased dopamine would serve to reduce her gross tremors. The goal was to monitor her behavior and to administer the medication as ordered. Nursing actions included the observation and reporting of any changes in behavior in addition to the administration of the drug. In the area of *reproduction,* Miss J. had no apparent problems. She was single, and her menstrual period was present and was normal. To facilitate normal functioning, the nursing action was to provide supplies as needed by the patient. Miss J. had no problem in relation to *body integrity* except allergy to soap. For this, she compensated by using a nonallergenic cleansing agent.

Psychosocial Needs

In the *psychological* area, it is conceivable that Miss J. may have been self-conscious about her poorly controlled movements, but this did not appear to be a great concern of hers. She had long since made the basic adjustment, and she would simply explain what she could and could not do so that other people could adjust their expectations of her. Miss J. was a college graduate with high honors, so the nursing staff provided psychological support by accepting her as a fully functioning person; also, they showed respect for her intelligence by giving full explanations that were geared to her level of understanding. In the *social area,* observation of her relationships with peers was difficult to obtain. None of her peers visited her during the author's observation. Miss J. gave the impression that she was highly independent except for the close associations with her parents and brother. The goal was to enhance her social interactions and to provide the climate for her optimum functioning. This was accomplished by increasing interaction with the patient and by allowing her adequate time to perform activities at her own pace. Encouraging other young people to interact with the patient was another nursing action.

In the areas of *culture and religion,* as Miss J. was Jewish, the goal was to respect and to consider her beliefs in planning diets and activities.

Nursing Concerns

In the area of *safety* of the patient, entropy was present in the form of her continuous gross movements that were mostly involuntary. Side effects of the drug levodopa represented another negative factor in the patient's safety. The safety goals were expressed by a need to safeguard her locomotion and to observe her closely for side effects of the drug as the dose was increased. The side effects of this drug can be many and varied, so any newly developed sensation or change in behavior should be noted and evaluated. In the area of *instruction,* as this patient was highly intelligent, it was simple to enhance her understanding of the therapy she was undergoing. The information was provided as she expressed a desire for it. In the coordination of this patient's care, the nurse was a liaison between the physician, the physical therapist, and the family. The goal was to facilitate communication in behalf of the patient. The completed assessment form inserted into the Kardex served as a prime source of communication regarding the patient's care needs.

In summary, the plan for Miss J.'s nursing care was as follows:

1. Encourage deep breathing and coughing
2. Monitor vital signs periodically
3. Encourage a high-caloric diet
4. Monitor bowel movements as necessary
5. Check and safeguard her hearing aid and speak slowly in front of her
6. Safeguard her locomotion and provide ample time for her to engage in her own activities
7. Supervise her exercises
8. Administer levodopa and observe effects
9. Accept her and respect her high intelligence
10. Consider her Jewish culture and religion
11. Attend to her safety from injury to herself
12. Instruct her in the side effects of the levodopa
13. Coordinate the efforts of the health team

The plan as derived above appears on page 66 in Table 8. This plan of care for Miss J. has been derived from an application of the concepts of general systems theory to the process of nursing assessment of patient care [1].

Another example of a nursing care plan and evaluation of nursing outcome based upon general systems theory has been developed by Ryan [2]. The reader is encouraged to compare formats.

References

1. Putt, A. M. Entropy, Evolution, and Equifinality in Nursing. In J. Smith (Ed.), *Five Years of Cooperation to Improve Curricula in Western Schools of Nursing.* Boulder, Colo.: Western Interstate Commission for Higher Education, 1972.
2. Ryan, B. Nursing care plans: A systems approach to developing criteria for planning and evaluation. *J. Nurs. Adm.* 3:(3)50, May–June, 1973.

Table 8. Nursing Care Plan – Miss J., Age 23

Area	Entropy (–) (Problems)	Evolution (+) (Resources)	Equifinality (Goal)	Nursing Action to Achieve Goal
Physiological needs				
Respiration	Athetoid respiration; weak cough	Continuous movement	Maintain	Encourage coughing and deep breathing
Circulation	Normal		Maintain	Monitor vital signs
Nutrition	Normal with excessive energy demands		Enhance	Give extra feedings, high-calorie diet
Elimination	Normal		Maintain	
Sensory perception	Nerve deafness	Hearing aid	Maintain	Speak slowly; protect hearing aid from damage
Locomotion	Continuous gross movements	PT exercises q.i.d.; has high intelligence	Maintain	Provide space and safety
Neuroendocrine	Severe cerebral palsy	Attempt at levodopa therapy		Explain procedure; monitor function
Body integrity	Allergic skin	Nonallergenic soap		Have nonallergic soap
Reproduction	Normal			Provide menstrual supplies as needed
Psychosocial needs				
Psychological	Self concept affected by C-P	High intelligence college graduate		Accept patient as a person; explain routines
Social	Few peers	Parents and brother attentive	Enhance	Encourage socialization
Religious		Jewish		Respect Jewish culture and beliefs
Nursing concerns				
Safety	Poorly controlled muscles; levodopa therapy	High intelligence	Expand	Observe; prevent injury
Instruction	Explain therapy		Expand knowledge	Instruct patient
Coordination of care		Patient responsible for most of her care	Maintain	Act as liaison for pt., family, Dr.

Name Miss J. Age 23 Room 8

Diagnosis Cerebral palsy Doctor Anderson

Source: The University of Arizona College of Nursing

Does Mr. C. Need a Care Plan?

8

Arlene M. Putt

"Nursing care plans are a snare and a delusion," declared Palisin [6, p. 63]. The author went on to say, "Nursing care plans are another communication burden imposed on the practitioner by the theorist.... It has been very fashionable to pick up cues, assess and plan – all this without getting validation from the patient himself about what is going on with him." Palisin's answer to better patient care is to do away with nursing care plans and to be more spontaneous and more highly individualized in nursing care. This approach, Palisin claimed, would further nursing service by freeing nurses from a large amount of paper work.

There are some serious flaws in this thinking. (1) Palisin assumes that nursing care plans are made without validating and revalidating the information with the patient. (2) The conclusion reached is based upon an unfounded assumption that the communication dilemma of the present-day hospital unit will be eased by less communication between individuals and fewer attempts at preserving the communication trace through written plans. Anyone cognizant of the present-day scene will recognize the multitudinous problems that exist now because communications by verbal channels *have* broken down; the solution to the dilemma is hardly more of the same.

A Cardiac Patient

What assistance would the use of the general systems theoretical framework provide the nurse faced with making a nursing care plan for a newly admitted patient? Let us look at the care of one cardiac patient.

The patient, Mr. C., is a 65-year-old retired bus driver who visited his physician because of chest pain. The pain was later described by the patient as sudden, severe midchest pain that radiated down both arms and up to the neck and jaw, causing mild sweating but no shortness of breath. His doctor prescribed a pain medication, name unknown by the patient, and sent Mr. C. home. The pain lasted one and one-half days. Over the next week, the patient had intermittent mild pain, but he remained at home on moderate-to-restricted activity. Four days prior to admission to the hospital, the patient again experienced severe pain that lasted 12 hours. He was again seen by his physician and again sent home with medication. The patient returned a third time in 3 more days; at this time an electrocardiogram (ECG) was taken, which showed a recent myocardial infarct. At this point, the patient was admitted to a general medical unit of a metropolitan hospital.

The physical examination on admission November 19 indicated the following: Mr. C. was an obese white male, aged 65, who smoked 1½ packs of cigarettes per day. He appeared flushed, with a blood pressure of 165/90, pulse 76, and respirations 16 per minute. There was mild arteriolar narrowing of the eye fundi, but no history of hypertension or diabetes mellitus. Bilaterally, Mr. C. had good carotid pulses with no bruits. His lungs were clear but emphysematous, with poor chest expansion. His heart sounds were distinct, with a normal pattern to sounds 1 and 2. There were no gallops and no definite murmurs. Mr. C.'s abdomen was obese but soft, with the liver 4 cm. below the umbilicus, and it was mildly tender but smooth. The spleen was not palpable. Both neurological and genital examinations showed normal findings, and Mr. C. had good pulses in the four extremities.

Mr. C.'s laboratory reports were as follows: hemoglobin 16.8 gm.; hematocrit 47 vol. per 100 ml.; total leukocytes 8,000 per cubic millimeter, with 65 segmented polymorphonuclear leukocytes, 4 eosinophils, 1 basophil, 21 lymphocytes, and 8 monocytes. The urinalysis showed negative findings. The creatine phosphokinase (CPK) was 11 units; the lactic dehydrogenase (LDH), 234; the serum glutamic-oxaloacetic transaminase (SGOT), 46; and the uric acid, 8.0 mg. The admission ECG showed Q waves in leads 2, 3, aVF, with ST depression in V_3 to V_6 and T wave inversion in leads 3 and aVF [5]. The ECG interpretation was that of a recent inferior infarct.

Mr. C. was ordered on bedrest with bathroom privileges, a 1,200-calorie diet, nitroglycerin 0.04 mg. p.r.n. for pain, and meperidine (Demerol) 50 mg. for pain that was unrelieved by nitroglycerin.

Nursing Care Without a Plan

Without a nursing care plan, each person concerned with Mr. C. must either read his chart to gather his own information or rely upon verbal and often casual comments of someone else. The latter is the more frequent choice of action. Many persons will contact Mr. C. during a week in the hospital. A minimum of six R.N.s will be his team leader for at least 8 hours. Many other persons such as licensed practical nurses, nurses' aides, interns, residents, orderlies, laboratory personnel, dietitians, dietary aides, ECG technicians, cleaning attendants, and even maintenance men may contact Mr. C. Are all these people going to depend upon word of mouth for information regarding Mr. C.? Are they all going to try to read his chart, or are they going to undertake their business without any information about this patient? Cleland [3] found that on a busy medical-surgical unit, registered nurses tended to respond to a very restricted range of information regarding any one patient and to record only the most obvious symptoms of the patient. Therefore, the supposed merit of each person gathering his own data regarding the patient is not very great.

What alternative exists? This author believes a practical solution lies in a short but systematic assessment made by the registered nurse [4]. Here the assessment is based on a triad of universal concepts that guides the processing of patient data into a sound prescription for nursing care. The process, utilizing Mr. C.'s care as an illustration, is described below.

Nursing Care With a Plan

First, let us assess Mr. C.'s biopsychosocial functioning at the present time. This can be done by considering the areas of respiration, circulation, nutrition, elimination, sensory perception, neuroendocrine integration, locomotion, body integrity, and reproduction. Assessment of his psychosocial functioning can be made by considering the psychological, social, cultural, and religious areas. Lastly, there are areas of nursing concern for the patient, namely, those of safety, instruction, and coordination of care. This format for outlining nursing care has been developed by the author from the work of von Bertalanffy [7] and Abbey [1].

Mr. C. has emphysema and has smoked 1½ packs of cigarettes per day for the past 50 years. This represents entropy in his respiratory functioning. Some evolutionary potential exists in his intention to give up smoking. The goal in relation to his respiration is to expand his ventilation, which may be achieved by the nurse's encouraging him to give up smoking, urging him to breathe deeply and slowly, and protecting him from dust. This patient's room in the hospital was located just a few feet away from a dusty service driveway. While his transfer to another bed may have been costly, since he had already been transferred from another nursing unit and had also had another bed on this unit, a third transfer might have been very desirable.

In the area of circulation, Mr. C. displayed his greatest entropy with the 2-week-old myocardial infarction; however, his coping ability was proving adequate, as he had not gone into shock and had not developed any arrhythmias. His resources were being conserved by bedrest with only bathroom privileges. The nursing goal for maintaining functioning was achieved by frequent observation of the patient's activity and his vital signs. With frequent observations, any changes could be promptly discerned and action could be taken.

Obesity represents another form of entropy and, in this patient, the obesity was counterbalanced by a 1,200-calorie diet with a restriction of the patient's usual beer intake. The goal was to reduce his weight, and the nurse acted by serving small meals designed to permit weight loss and prevent gastric distention against impaired heart muscle. Also, the nurse checked the patient's intake and weighed the patient frequently.

Mr. C.'s elimination was normal, but straining was to be prevented by intake of laxative foods such as prune juice. The nursing action was to check the patient's functioning daily and administer a laxative if the patient needed it.

Mr. C. had normal sensory perception except for requiring glasses for reading; however, his locomotion was greatly restricted because of his cardiac impairment. The goal was to restrict his locomotion until his heart had an opportunity to heal. He was confined to 5 days of bedrest with only bathroom privileges.

His neuroendocrine, his body integrity, and his reproductive functioning were normal and did not require further consideration at this time.

In the psychosocial realm, Mr. C. was married to a woman approximately 15 years younger who was of Mexican-American descent. They had two teenage daughters. The family was active in the Catholic church. Mr. C. has always been the breadwinner of the family and he did not want his wife to work, but since his retirement, his health had not permitted his working so the family was living on social security benefits. Mr. C. owned a house trailer with two rooms attached; it was located on an unpaved street at the southwest edge of the city. The family did not have a phone. As a group, the family members were very close and supportive of each other; the parents spent much time with their children, and the girls gave evidence of respecting and obeying their parents. Frequently, the family took camping trips in another small sport trailer. While the myocardial infarct was a threat to Mr. C.'s independence and position as head of the family, the solidarity of the family support and their involvement were assets in his ability to cope with the illness.

For the safety of Mr. C., his smoking in bed and his acceptance of his limited activity were factors to be considered. His environment was made safe by prohibiting his smoking in bed, discouraging his smoking elsewhere, and limiting his activity to his tolerance and orders. Mr. C., while not a highly educated man, was average or above average in intelligence, and so it was possible to explain and reenforce his understanding of his illness and his restrictions. The family was included in this instruction, and they also served to reenforce it. The patient's coordination of care required planning with the family and with his various doctors. A total of four cardiologists read Mr. C.'s series of ECGs, and the impressions differed slightly as to the area of involvement. His family physician needed to be included in his discharge plans. Basically, one concern here was not to discontinue this patient's care upon his discharge from the hospital, but rather to provide follow-up care at home.

Summary

In summary, the nursing care plan was developed with Mr. C. and revolved around concern for his impaired cardiac function, his need to limit dietary intake and activity, and his psychological need for support during a threatening illness. While these needs are not unique to this patient, the assessment of the patient was made from his unique constellation of needs and provided full coverage of his functioning. Therefore, the plan of care was not imposed *upon* Mr. C., but rather developed *with* him. This plan is summarized in Table 9.

Does Mr. C. Need a Care Plan?

Table 9. Nursing Care Plan – Mr. C., Age 65

Area	Entropy (–) (Problems)	Evolution (+) (Resources)	Equifinality (Goal)	Nursing Action to Achieve Goal
Physiological needs				
Respiration	Smokes 1½ pk/day Emphysema	His goal no smoking	Enhance ventilation	Encourage no smoking; urge deep slow breathing; protect from dust
Circulation	2-week-old infarction	No CHF or arrhythmia	Maintain	Observe patient and vital signs
Nutrition	Obese	1,200-cal. diet	Limit	Restrict beer; prescribe small meals
Elimination	Normal	Laxative foods	Maintain	Monitor, discourage straining
Sensory perception	Reading glasses		Maintain	
Locomotion	2-week MI	Bedrest/BRP	Restrict	Monitor activity
Neuroendocrine			Maintain	
Body integrity			Maintain	
Reproduction			Restrict temporarily	
Psychosocial needs				
Psychological	Retired; ego-threatening illness	Strong determination	Enhance	Encourage patient
Social/Cultural	Retired	Wife and 2 daughters, Mexican-American	Maintain	Include family
Religious		Catholic	Maintain	
Nursing concerns				
Safety	Smokes; pushes activity		Enhance	Prohibit smoking Limit activity
Instruction		Average intelligence	Enhance	Instruct patient and family re: healing, diet, activity
Coordination of care	Multiple MDs		Maintain	Coordinate hospital-home, multiple MDs

Name Mr. C. Age 65 Room 13

Diagnosis Inferior myocardial infarction Doctor Larkin

Source: The University of Arizona College of Nursing

Mr. C.'s progress was as follows: his CPK value went from 11 to 8; his LDH from 234 to 148; his SGOT went from 46 to 32; and his uric acid went from 8.0 to 8.3 mg. percent. On his 1,200-calorie diet, his weight went from 168 to 163 pounds. During 5 days of bedrest with bathroom privileges, Mr. C. showed no arrhythmias or signs of congestive failure; however, Mr. C. did have difficulty in restricting himself to his limited activity. When he was permitted out of bed, he took walks in the hall. These walks were followed in 2 to 3 hours by prolonged bouts of angina, a repeated occurrence well documented in the nurses' notes. While this activity did not produce an extension of the infarct, the ECG demonstrated persistent ischemia. On admission, Mr. C.'s ECG had shown first-degree heart block and possible inferior myocardial infarction. After a series of ECGs, the interpretation of December 7 was the change since November 19 had been little and not characteristic of the usual evolutionary changes one would expect 2½ weeks after infarct. The conclusion was that the ECGs would have to be interpreted with the clinical and laboratory picture of the patient.

During his stay in the hospital, Mr. C. was told of the death of a brother-in-law. This he accepted without distress. He told one nurse that he did not know his brother-in-law very well and so the death did not put a strain on him.

After a postponement of 5 days, the patient was discharged, on December 11, doing well. His doctor directed him to remain inactive for one month and then gradually to resume his activities. The medication he took home was isosorbide dinitrate (Isordil Tembids), 40 mg. twice a day (b.i.d.). This drug acts as a nitrite and is intended for the prophylaxis of angina pectoris.

Readjustment of this patient's care plan would have entailed the following: First, ideally, this patient should have been admitted to the hospital earlier in the course of his illness. Also, the two transfers, because of disturbances by roommates, might have been avoided. Locating the patient next to a dusty driveway was unwise because of his emphysema. Some of his bouts of angina could have been prevented by restricting his activity more; however, the patient was resistive to limited activity. He had a deep need to prove to himself that he could be active with no ill effects. Intermittent instruction regarding the need for restricted activity did not change his behavior. He continued to press his limits and to prove to himself what he could and could not do. This was one of the reasons for following Mr. C. after discharge. The plan for Mr. C. would be readjusted after the first home visit.

Posthospital Care

The first home visit was made 4 days after discharge. Mr. C.'s house trailer is located in a fenced yard about 25 feet from a very dusty and heavily traveled unpaved street. There is a thick layer of light brown dust over the yard and the trees; this is added to with each passing car. Mrs. C. answered the door. The patient was dressed and sitting in a chair with his feet elevated, watching television. He had had no further chest pain and was asking about the possibility of increasing his activity. To answer some of his questions, the booklet "After a Coronary" [2] was given to him, with some clarification. Mr. C.'s wife and daughters were very supportive toward him and the wife demonstrated that she had good control over him without appearing to dominate him. Mr. C. had lost 4 more pounds and was adhering to his diet; however, he complained of food sticking in his throat. This he was encouraged to discuss with his family physician when he returned for a visit the following week. At this time, a readjusted plan of care based upon his previous plan was made.

A visit was attempted right after Christmas, but the patient was asleep and was not seen.

By December 29, Mr. C. was doing well. He was down to 158 pounds and had had no discomfort since his early walking periods. His family physician had extended his activity, and he was now walking three-quarters of a mile 3 times a day. On this day, his intention was to increase his walking for a fourth time for a total of 3 miles a day. He was cautioned about cold and windy weather and instructed not to get overly tired in his attempts to increase his endurance.

By the next visit, on January 6, the temperature had been down to 18°–20°F for three mornings. The patient had walked 7 miles on Saturday, but decided that 6 miles would have been a better amount. Since then, the weather had been cold, and he said that he did not mind the walking, but that the inhalation of cold air hurt his chest and gave him a sense of heaviness; therefore, he had discontinued walking until the weather warmed. He felt that he could resume walking when the temperature reached 50°F. His weight was still 158 pounds. He had had more difficulty in his swallowing, and he had discussed this with his doctor, who wished to wait another few weeks before checking out his complaint. According to the patient, food of any kind appeared to stick about one-third of the way down the esophagus. At times, even water stopped there and was regurgitated. On questioning, he said he had not had this difficulty before his illness. He was urged to consult the doctor again and he said he would.

During the January 15 visit, two months after infarct, the outdoor temperature was 60°F and the patient was out walking for 40 minutes. This was the nurse's first opportunity to talk with his wife alone. She said he had not complained of further difficulty in swallowing, and he had not returned to the doctor as yet. He was due to return in about two more weeks. His wife reported that he had lost another 2 pounds. The main problem now was that the patient was getting irritable with his daughters for no obvious reason. This was explored more fully and possible explanations were reviewed. Also, the topic of dust was brought into the conversation. The street situation was very bad and no relief was in sight. Mr. C. had discussed moving out of town to a lot that a relative owns in a small town about 80 miles away. The older daughter was resistant to this idea, for she wished to go to college while living at home, so this decision remained open. At this point in the conversation, the patient had returned from his walk, tired but rosy. He appeared to be getting impatient with convalescence, and he may have been withholding information as to how he really felt. He asked how long it would take before full recovery was reached. He was told that 6 to 9 months was not unusual for the maximum return of activity. The patient appeared much thinner, and gave the impression that he was more concerned about his future than he was saying. Further follow-up was made.

On February 3, an attempt was made to visit the patient, but he was not home.

On February 4, the patient was passed in a car en route to having x-rays and laboratory studies. By stopping to converse briefly, the following information was obtained. Mr. C. had been short of breath. He had been back to the doctor and was having laboratory studies performed. The swallowing problem was not too bad, but the shortness of breath did bother him. Mr. C. did not feel that the shortness of breath was caused by the dust storm and the 46-mile-per-hour winds of the previous day. An appointment was made to visit the patient at home on February 22. He had been rechecked by the physician in the meantime, and an upper gastrointestinal x-ray series had been done, with a favorable report. Mr. C. was still experiencing shortness of breath at night. He had been started on digoxin (Lanoxin), 0.25 mg. daily, and his wife took his pulse daily. He was back to walking 3½ miles per day. Mr. C. said he felt better after he had started walking again; however, he had not walked that day. His weight was stable at 156 pounds. The action of the digoxin was reviewed with both the patient and his wife.

On March 11, the patient was now doing well, except for bleeding gums. He was taking sodium warfarin (Coumadin), 5 mg. daily. The need to see a dentist and why this was important in view of his medication was discussed at length. Mr. C. said he was not eligible for care at the County Hospital, so the County had given him a letter of referral to a free clinic. He was urged to try this source for dental care or to visit a private dentist at least once. A discussion of the situation at the time of his primary illness indicated that he had not gone to the hospital when he first became ill because this occurred one month before he would have been 65 years of age, and he could not afford a hospital bill at that time. He had waited until Medicare would pay his bill. Mr. C.'s weight was stable, and he was working around the yard rather than walking.

On April 1, it was learned that the patient was having paroxysmal nocturnal dypsnea (PND) that got him up and walking at 4 A.M. His doctor suggested a wedge for his bed, and he was now using this device under the head of the bed with some effect. Mr. C. was urged to cut his salt intake. Salt intake had been discussed with him previously, but he continued to salt his food heavily. He had not been back to the doctor; however, both of his cats had been seriously ill with some kind of distemper, and *they* had been taken to the veterinarian several times. In addition, both daughters and his wife had had the flu. Mr. C. continued to take the sodium warfarin and digoxin, but he had not yet seen a dentist. The importance of adequate health care for him was again stressed.

On April 22, the patient was still having PND. Again, he was urged to decrease his salt intake. To this point, he had been noncooperative, but he said perhaps he would comply this time. Mr. C. had not been to the dentist yet, so the importance of receiving treatment for his bleeding gums was again stressed.

Does Mr. C. Need a Care Plan?

Mr. C. was now talking about going to Arkansas for the summer. He had no daytime discomfort and was able to work around the yard and the trailer. His weight remained stable.

On May 20, the visit to Mr. C. was not made until late afternoon. Because he had no phone, he could not be told of the change in time. He had wondered why the visit had not been made at the usual time. At this point, his PND was better. He had cut his salt intake and agreed that food now tasted better. Mr. C. still had not been to see either the doctor or the dentist. He had decided not to go to Arkansas because the distance was too far. Also, his older daughter was starting as a candy striper in June. The family planned to go to the mountains for a trip. Mr. C. looked good and said that he felt good, also. One more nursing visit was planned for during the summer.

On May 31, the older daughter called early in the morning to say that her father had dropped dead on May 28. He had taken the trailer to a lake site about 70 miles away, with the rest of the family following a few hours later in the car. This was his first camping trip. When the family got there, he rose to greet them and motioned where they were to park. Before they could get the leashes on the cats, he sat down on the trailer steps and the younger daughter saw him fall backward. He died immediately. Mr. C. was given mouth-to-mouth resuscitation, and was taken to the nearest hospital 30 miles away but was dead on arrival. The autopsy report indicated massive infarct and extensive arteriosclerosis. The body was returned to the city and burial was delayed until the end of the week. Relatives gathered and the family appeared composed.

A nursing visit was made before the funeral. The extended family was in attendance. Mrs. C.'s mother, an elderly Mexican woman who spoke only Spanish, had arrived. Numerous in-laws and siblings were taking turns staying with the family. Mrs. C. was still in the shock phase, but she said that it was a comfort to have her family at hand. She was having guilty feelings about allowing her husband to drive the trailer that day and about the rest of the family not getting to the lake sooner. A relative had met Mr. C. on the way to the campsite and had stopped to chat. Mr. C. appeared fine at that point. Mrs. C. was allowed to express her grief and guilt feelings, and the fact that this could have happened at any time or place was pointed out to her. The fact that the patient had died a quick and happy death gave her some degree of comfort. The nurse said she would like to attend the funeral, and Mrs. C. said that she thought Mr. C. would have appreciated that. She thanked her sincerely for coming.

On June 3, a visit was made to view Mr. C. at the funeral home. At that time, none of the family was in attendance.

The funeral mass was attended on June 4, after which the trip to the cemetery was made across town. The family was in deep grief, but received understanding and kind support from their relatives. The younger daughter turned to the nurse at the grave-side. The family appreciated the nurse's willingness to go all the way.

On June 22, a visit was again made to the family, and the events leading up to Mr. C.'s death were discussed with less intensity. Mrs. C.'s feelings of guilt were still present, but discussing this freely allowed her to work through her feelings.

 Continuing emotional support was offered. The family was planning on having a telephone installed; this will of course facilitate closer contact with the family. The older daughter had become a candy striper and was busy with these activities.

Telephone contacts were maintained throughout the summer. About once a week, either the girls or their mother would call, or a call would be made to them. Mrs. C. was ill about a month after the funeral. She had several teeth that were badly decayed and also had pyorrhea. She, too, was urged to make an appointment at the clinic, and she indicated that she would.

On August 1, two months after the funeral, the nurse provided the family with a picnic as a change of pace.

Contact by phone was continued. In early September, Mrs. C. was again very ill because of her teeth. She finally had made a dental appointment, but the pain was so severe that she had to go earlier than her appointment. The dentist's one concern was why she had not come sooner. He extracted two teeth and planned to fill another one and extract two other teeth. The week after this, the younger daughter had a severe infection that required a doctor's visit and antibiotics. A possible relation to the pyorrhea was questioned.

On October 9, the girls called. The older daughter and the mother had "stomach flu," which they believed they got from an uncle. The younger daughter recovered from her infection and did not get the flu. Mrs. C. had another dental appointment scheduled for October 20. The older daughter had heard of Med Start and wanted to explore this possible opportunity. At the end of an 11-month sequence of events, the family was continuing their readjustment process, and the wife was starting to think about employment to supplement their income from social security.

"Cardiac nursing, general systems style" in this author's terms means a continuing concern and follow-up of the patient. The patient with myocardial infarction, such as Mr. C., is not functioning at his fullest when he leaves the hospital. He needs someone to follow his progress at home and to correlate his hospital and home experiences. Neither the hospital nurse who sees the patient only in the hospital, nor the public health nurse who sees the patient only in the home setting can do this follow-up with any continuity or understanding. What the answer is to this dilemma and division of care is not clear. Surely the dichotomizing of care into episodic and distributive aspects hardly seems to be an answer. Mr. C. needed care that extended over seven months and two settings.

Mr. C. is one of many thousands of patients who have received fractionated care under the present system for delivery of health services. The health delivery system could be adapted to provide better care in a more coordinated fashion by universal utilization of a consistent appraisal and progress form. The development and use of such a tool comprise the challenge before the health professions and the nation at this time. A general systems approach to nursing care plans could be utilized to help bridge the gap between phases of health care.

References

1. Abbey, J. A General Systems Approach to Nursing. In J. Smith (Ed.), *Improvement of Curricula in Schools of Nursing.* Boulder, Colo.: Western Interstate Commission for Higher Education, 1970.
2. American Heart Association. *After a Coronary.* New York: American Heart Association, 1970.
3. Cleland, V. S. Effects of stress on thinking. *Am. J. Nurs.* 67:108, 1967.
4. Glover, M. *A Systematic Approach to the Nursing Care Plan.* New York: Appleton-Century-Croft, 1972.
5. Goldman, M. J. *Principles of Clinical Electrocardiography* (7th ed.). Los Altos, Calif.: Lange Medical Publications, 1970.
6. Palisin, H. E. Nursing care plans are a snare and a delusion. *Am. J. Nurs.* 71:63, 1971.
7. von Bertalanffy, L. *General System Theory.* New York: George Braziller, 1968.

Tools for Teaching 9

I. General Systems Theory Nursing Care Plans

Arlene M. Putt

Nursing care plans written according to the general systems format provide excellent tools for teaching [2]. The plans are useful to help students and staff do the following:

1. Think in a logical manner
2. Gather pertinent data systematically
3. Take responsibility for individual interpretation and actions
4. Formulate goals appropriate to the patient's situation
5. Select actions to achieve the selected goals
6. Evaluate the outcomes of the nursing actions
7. Guide the learning of pathophysiology
8. Set priorities for care to patients
9. Strive toward total individualized care for patients
10. Organize information for charting and reporting
11. Encourage constant updating of the care plans
12. Learn reversible from irreversible processes occurring in the patients
13. Recognize the development of evolutionary happenings that signal progress and growth in the patients
14. Anticipate the outcomes of increasing entropies observable in the patients
15. Recognize the consequences of poor care and analyze where the process went astray
16. Utilize the plans as models of care to be achieved
17. Utilize the care plans as the basis for nursing conferences and interdisciplinary team conferences

While this list appears long, it is not exhaustive. As these uses are discussed more fully, additional uses will probably occur to the reader.

Thinking in a logical manner is one of the prime requisites for any person involved in the delivery of health care. Unless thinking is practiced in a systematic way, chaos soon reigns. The professional health worker must learn to think logically and objectively about the multiple situations that are encountered in the course of professional activities. If, early in their studies, health workers learn a systematic framework for thinking and practice its use, thought processes can become habitual. However, the resulting thought is still complete and logically organized. It is hoped that there will be some transference of this thinking format to other similar endeavors.

Gathering pertinent data is greatly facilitated when the outline calls attention to what data are needed and when the outline proceeds in some sort of a systematic manner from one topic to another until the entire body of information is covered.

A professional must take responsibility for individual interpretation and individual actions. Also, the professional accepts responsibility for interpretation and judgment-making with a sense of accountability and pride. If the process were totally automatic, there would be no challenge in it. In nursing, the challenge of unique individuals encountering rapidly changing and very variable situations is always present. If the professional is tuned to respond to this challenge, a high quality of health care results. If the challenge is avoided, routinization sets in and depersonalization occurs.

Formulating goals appropriate to the patient's situation necessitates a certain level of knowledge as to what is appropriate for the patient. Where knowledge is adequate, this setting of goals is processed easily. Where knowledge is inadequate, additional counsel or knowledge must be sought prior to the determination of the goals or after a trial. The development of a less desirable situation indicates that the goal was inappropriate for the patient in that particular situation. Recognizing the need for more knowledge and seeking that needed knowledge are parts of the ongoing process of learning to be a professional.

The evaluation of the outcomes of selected actions is the feedback process that is necessary for restructuring plans and for correcting errors. If one action does not appear to improve the situation, it should be reconsidered and another approach selected. Through this process, the options available are gradually learned and the experienced person has additional methods that can be tried in turn.

Learning pathophysiology is inherent in learning to provide high-quality health care. One cannot plan appropriate care if one does not understand the nature and degree of the processes that have been disrupted. Because of the rapid increase in the body of available knowledge, an individual's understanding of any one topic is subject to repeated challenge. Therefore, constant effort must be made to keep abreast of the understanding of the patient's disorder and the possible approaches to correcting the dysfunction.

Setting priorities for care is a necessary skill needed all too frequently when the demands in the situation exceed the resources of the staff to meet the needs. Some matters are more pressing than others. Therefore, learning which matters require top priority, and when top priority is essential to getting urgent matters attended to in time to change the course of events becomes very important.

Total individualized care to patients is a goal given frequent lip service with less attention in the real life situation. The general systems theory approach to health care facilitates attention to this aspect of service. By gathering data systematically from the patient, the nurse learns to know the patient as an individual with a unique constellation of problems in varying degree. Working out a plan of care for the patient becomes a realization of the individuality that has become apparent during the interaction. This is a point where instruction can point out crucial differences that may have been overlooked.

Organizing information for reports and charting is easily accomplished when the outline is before the worker to remind him what areas of information should be reviewed and considered for additional comment. By cross-checking the reports with the general systems care plan, any area of omission can easily be detected and corrected.

Updating plans recorded in pencil is easily accomplished, especially when the plans are reviewed with each change of responsibility and at each nursing report. To maintain a record of previous information, the method of drawing red lines through data no longer of use can be helpful. Thus, if the situation fluctuates back and forth, the previous methods are still available. Also, outcomes can more easily be traced to the methods that produced them.

Learning to differentiate reversible from irreversible processes that are occurring in patients is another professional skill that has to be learned by experience. By focusing upon the degree and rate of change of the various entropies in the patient, this learning is more easily acquired.

Learning to recognize and to capitalize upon the positive happenings that show progress and growth in a healthy direction is still another professional judgment that must be developed. This development is facilitated by attention to the changes that are occurring in this aspect, to the rate of the change, and to the resources that have been brought to bear upon the patient's situation.

By identifying the entropies as they occur and possibly develop, the nurse becomes prepared for the inescapable outcome. If the system is stressed beyond its resiliency, collapse of the system can be anticipated and supportive measures begun, or else the death of the patient can be expected. By noting the changes as they occur, the nurse can learn where death begins and whether there is merit in fighting death or accepting it. Thus, the nurse learns to better understand the process of dying.

With the built-in evaluation and reassessment, identifying unsatisfactory outcomes should be easy to achieve. Reworking the assessment and decision-making processes should leave clues as to why the process went astray. Then the faulty processes can be adjusted so desired outcomes are more likely to be achieved in the future. Here again, instruction can guide the restructuring process.

One large area for using general systems theory care plans as a teaching tool is to use them as models of standards of care. With models as guides, it is easier to achieve a given level of quality of nursing care [1]. Given the present emphasis on standardized nursing care plans, the general systems theory format is ideal. With model plans available beforehand, less time is needed to adjust plans to individual needs.

Finally, care plans using this base can be used as teaching tools in every nursing report and team conference. With more well-organized information immediately available, there is more to report and to discuss. In interdisciplinary team conferences, each discipline can find one or more areas in which complementary information or services can be included so that the overall care is improved.

Thus, the reader can see multiple teaching uses for this care plan and compare it with other plans [1].

References

1. Carter, J. H., Hilliard, M., Castles, M., Stoll, L., and Coor, A. *Standard of Nursing Care: A Guide for Evaluation.* New York: Springer Publishing, 1976.
2. Ryan, B. J. Nursing care plans: A systems approach to developing criteria for planning and evaluation. *J. Nurs. Adm.* 3:(3)50, May–June, 1973.

II. Design for a Clinical Nursing Course

Ellen Kval Isaak

Nursing IIA, Clinical Nursing in Acute, Disruptive Conditions, is an eight-credit course offered during the second semester of the junior year. The nursing curriculum for which this course is developed is built on two years of intensive study in the biological, physical and social sciences. This provides an academic background of 66 to 70 credits to enable the student to integrate the cognitive, psychomotor and affective domains necessary in nursing [1].

Nursing courses account for 57 units of the 135 to 140 units of credit necessary for a baccalaureate degree. General systems theory provides the framework for the curriculum. Emphasizing man in his biopsychosocial entirety, the holistic approach to nursing covers man's adaptation from conception to death, from wellness to illness, through varying levels of health care involving individuals and groups [4]. The nursing process is the strand of knowledge and practice throughout the curriculum and underscores the integrative nature of nursing content. Accountability, leadership, assessment and management are interdependent and all courses stress primary care nursing [2]. Adhering to the concept of continuous progress and mastery learning, nursing courses are all interrelated. While research is an integral part of the curriculum, the major emphasis on research is reserved for the senior year.

After the two years of initial preparation, the course, Nursing IIA, is designed to build on a foundation established in ten credits of nursing, four credits of pharmacy and three credits of nutrition. In this course communication skills are expanded and the relationships of concepts and decision-making processes become more complex. Emphasizing the adult patient, Nursing IIA is taken concurrently with Nursing IIB, Maternal-Child Nursing, six credits, and Biochemistry, three credits. Recognizing certain concepts are universal throughout nursing, content for the nursing courses is complementary [3] (Fig. 5).

Note: This section describes a hypothetical course designed as part of a projected nursing curriculum based on general systems theory.

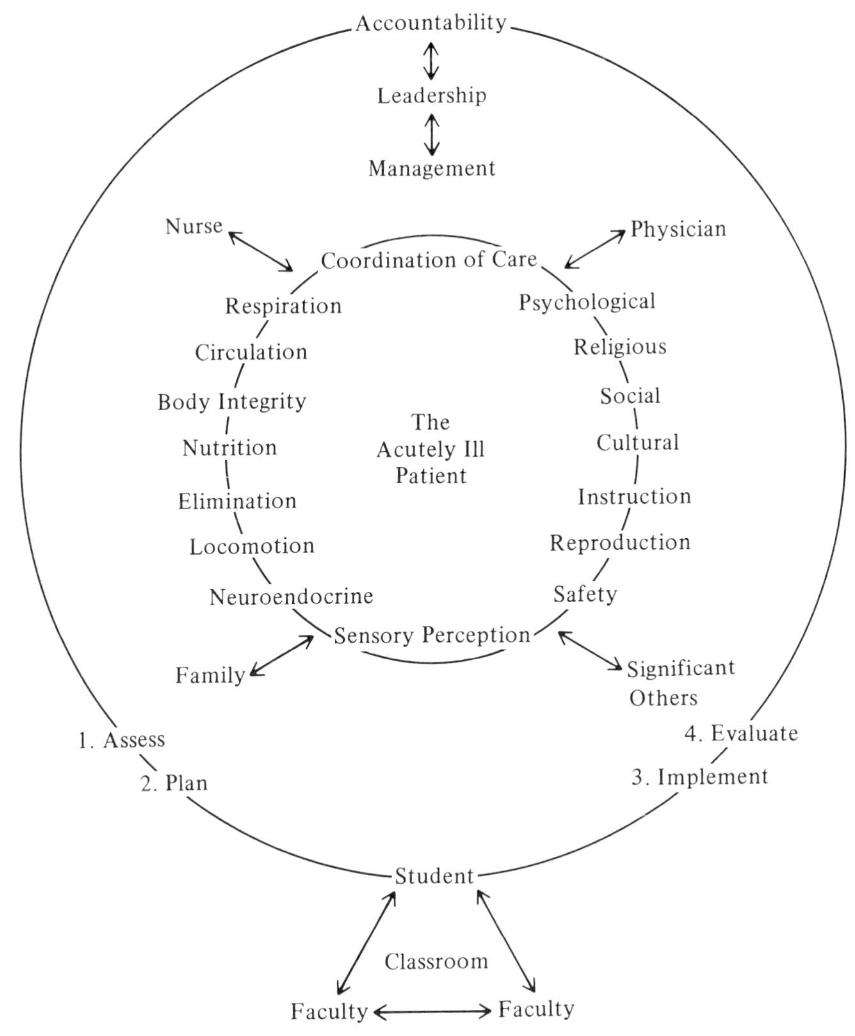

Figure 5. A model for a nursing course.

Supervised clinical practice is correlated with classroom material [3]. Clinical practice will be obtained on general medical and surgical units of an acute care institution. Each clinical laboratory group is limited to eight students who have rotating experiences lasting five weeks each.

Course Objectives

Upon completion of this course, the student will be able to do the following:

1. Utilize the nursing process in the nursing care of the acutely ill medical-surgical patient
   a. Assess the biopsychosocial needs of the patient

   b. Plan the nursing interventions to meet the needs of the patient
   c. Implement the nursing interventions by direct patient care (physical and emotional)
   d. Evaluate the effectiveness of the nursing interventions
2. Synthesize knowledge from the physical and social sciences as a basis for making nursing decisions
   a. Increase knowledge of normal physiology by recognizing pathophysiology
   b. Recognize psychosocial and cultural aspects of patient needs
   c. Apply nutrition principles to meet patient needs
   d. Apply pharmacological principles to patient care
3. Utilize known nursing interventions obtained through review of the literature
   a. Relate rationale for nursing interventions
   b. Analyze biopsychosocial effects of nursing interventions
   c. Plan and implement nursing care based on scientific principles
4. Analyze pathophysiological needs of the patient using physical assessment skills as an objective tool on which to base nursing interventions
   Demonstrate skill in physical assessment through (1) interviewing, (2) auscultation, (3) percussion, (4) palpation, (5) inspection
5. Share in the responsibility for the health and welfare of the patient and his family with other members of the health team
   a. Be accountable for all nursing actions taken while providing patient care
   b. Participate in team conferences
   c. Teach and/or counsel the patient and/or his family
   d. Initiate primary, secondary, and tertiary nursing interventions
6. Identify with the role of change agent in dealing with the patient, adhering to the components of primary nursing care
   a. Demonstrate leadership in patient advocacy and meeting the needs and goals of the patient
   b. Manage patient care by coordinating the health care provided to the patient
   c. Utilize self-assessment in evaluating effectiveness of nursing actions
   d. Utilize self-assessment in evaluating learning needs to further educational goals

Grading

Course grading will be as follows.

Theory	40%	Two major examinations	20%
		One final examination	15%
		One term paper	5%
Clinical	60%	Performance	50%
		Health assessment paper	10%

	Monday	Wednesday	Friday
Physiological needs			
Week 1 Respiration	Introduction Dynamics of ventilation/respiration Defense mechanisms Gas exchange	Physical assessment: thorax and lungs; chest tubes	Acute respiratory disorders Asthma, COPD, tuberculosis
Week 2 Circulation	Circulatory dynamics Hematologic disorders Heart failure Cardiopulmonary resuscitation	Physical assessment: cardiovascular system Basic ECG interpretation	ASHD, hypertension, CAD, myocardial infarction
Week 3 Elimination	Renal dynamics Renal disorders and renal failure	Physical assessment: integumentary system Ostomy care	Acid-base balance: fluid and electrolytes
Week 4 Nutrition	Gastrointestinal dynamics Absorption disturbances Liver function	Physical assessment: abdomen. Gavage/lavage IVAC/IMED	Special diets: ulcer, sodium-restricted, Fad diets
Week 5 Body integrity	Concepts of auto-immunity Rheumatoid arthritis	Physical assessment: extremities and back Aids in ADL	Altered body image Rehabilitation/Habilitation
Week 6 Locomotion	Examination	Review of exam	Musculoskeletal disorders Osteoporosis Fractures
Week 7 Neurological	Neurological overview Parkinson's Unconscious patient	Physical assessment: neurological Circo-Electric Stryker frame	Spinal cord injuries Paraplegia (term paper due)
Week 8 Endocrinology	Concepts of endocrinology Pituitary, thyroid, adrenals	Diagnostic procedures Analyzing laboratory data	Diabetes
Week 9 Sensory perception	Disorders of the eye and ear Aphasia	Physical assessment: eye, ear, nose, and throat	Sleep Sensory deprivation Sensory overload (health assessment due)
Psychosocial needs			
Week 10 Psychological	Concept of pain	Physical assessment: mental status Diagnostic procedures EMI/Scans	Psychosomatic disorders

	Monday	Wednesday	Friday
Psychosocial needs (Cont.)			
Week 11 Reproduction	Examination	Review of examination	Human sexuality
Week 12 Sociological	Concept of anxiety	Discussion of privacy/ patient advocacy	Addiction Hospital drug problems
Week 13 Cultural/ Religion	Grief and mourning Death and dying	Discussion of student views Role-playing	Local cultural beliefs (Mexican, Indian, Black, low socioeconomic groups)
Nursing concerns			
Week 14 Instruction	Principles of teaching/ learning theories	Patient teaching Discharge planning	Nursing audit Quality assurance
Week 15 Safety	Hospital-acquired illnesses Architectural barriers	Awareness session (student experiences, simulated handicaps)	Communicable diseases

*Supervised clinical practice will be correlated with lecture and seminar material.

References

1. Bigge, M. L. *Learning Theories for Teachers* (3d ed.). New York: Harper & Row, 1976.
2. McGivern, D. O., Mezey, M. D., and Baer, E. D. Teaching primary care in a baccalaureate program. *Nurs. Outlook* 24:441–445, 1976.
3. Miller, Sister P. Clinical knowledge: A needed curriculum emphasis. *Nurs. Outlook* 23:222–224, 1975.
4. Roy, Sister C. Adaptation: Implications for curriculum change. *Nurs. Outlook* 21:163–168, 1973.

General Systems Theory Nursing Care Plans: Long Forms

10

The general systems theory nursing care plan is versatile, as it can be adapted to whatever degree of precision is desired. If students are using it to learn about pathophysiology, the entropy column in the form used can be as detailed as desired, with as much information as can be obtained on each and every aspect of entropy in each system and subsystem. In this case, a long format develops. If the plan is intended for the busy nursing staff on the unit, many of whom are aides, the detailed accounts of pathophysiological conditions may not be appropriate and so a much shorter and simpler format can be devised (Chap. 11). The reader can decide how much information is desirable in any one situation. There is no hard and fast rule to follow. Adaptation to the situation at hand is the key.

I. A Patient with Guillain-Barré Syndrome

Roberta Ann Palmer

Mrs. E. C., a 68-year-old woman with Guillain-Barré syndrome, was admitted to the hospital in March 1976. She was obese and bedridden. Her speech was slurred but she was alert and responded appropriately.

The onset of the syndrome occurred about a month prior to her admission. It followed flu-like symptoms and a cough [1, 2].

The diagnosis was as follows: Guillain-Barré syndrome; chronic bronchitis; flu-like symptoms associated with the onset of Guillain-Barré syndrome; malignant hypertension of 6 years duration – controlled medically; arteriosclerotic heart disease and angina pectoris; history of transient ischemic attacks (TIA); Bell's palsy associated with onset of Guillain-Barré syndrome [3]; symptomatic osteoarthritis with deformity – Heberden's nodes and hip pain; chronic obesity; and elevated blood sugar with a family history of diabetes mellitus.

The patient, a Protestant, lives in a community in northern Arizona with her husband, son, and daughter-in-law. She has a sister who also lives in Arizona. Her husband is a middle-class retiree and she is insured by Medicare.

Medications given were dioctyl sodium sulfosuccinate (Colace), 100 mg. (q.d.); hydrochlorothiazide (Hydrodiuril), 100 mg. (every AM); methyl-dopate (Aldomet), 500 mg. (t.i.d.); digoxin 0.125 mg. (q.d.); amitriptyline (Elavil), 50 mg. (q.d.); potassium chloride (KCL), 20 mEq. (t.i.d.); and acetaminophen (Tylenol) and milk of magnesia (p.r.n.).

Mrs. E. C.'s symptoms gradually improved, and in time she gained increased strength in the distal muscles. She did not require a tracheotomy and the palsy symptoms were resolved.

Table 10. Nursing Care Plan (Long Form) – Mrs. E. C., Age 68*

Area	Entropy (–) (Problems)	Evolution (+) (Resources)	Equifinality	Nursing Action
Physiological needs				
Respiration	Chronic bronchitis for 2 yr. Flu-like symptoms (with cough) since February (probably coincides with onset of Guillain-Barré syndrome). →↑ leukocytes in response to infection; possible evolving respiratory failure from paralysis of respiratory musculature caused by progression of ascending paralysis of Guillain-Barré syndrome; chest x-ray of Mar. 17 shows infiltrate → possible lower lobe pneumonitis from ↓ cough reflex → inability to move accumulated secretions from chronic infection or from aspiration pneumonia owing to ↓ swallowing reflex	↑ Improvement of pulmonary function tests since admission; no sign of respiratory depression or distress and ascending paralysis is subsiding; abnormally high leukocyte count on admission now normal	Prevention of further complications from underlying respiratory infection; maintain optimal respiratory functioning through course of disease; clear chest x-ray	1. Observe patient (pt.) carefully for signs of respiratory depression or distress 2. Keep tracheotomy tray and suction equipment at bedside 3. Monitor results of pulmonary function tests for ↓ forced vital capacity (FVC), and forced expiratory volume (FEV) 4. Monitor temperature for ↑ significant of ↑ respiratory infection 5. Listen for adventitious breath sounds 6. Turn frequently to prevent stasis pneumonia 7. Prevent aspiration pneumonia by feeding small amounts of liquid slowly, with nurse in attendance throughout feeding
Circulation	Malignant hypertension for 6 yr. – highest BP 208/110; accelerated hypertension →↑ renal damage → possibility of eventual renal failure and death if not controlled ↓	Hypertension controlled with methyldopate, spironolactone (Aldactazide), and hydrochlorothiazide BP 180-185/90-95; only slight retinal changes and no retinal exudates	Maintain BP	1. Make frequent BP checks as current disease may cause exacerbation 2. Watch potassium (K^+) levels as pt. is on heavy load of diuretics; K^+ supplements

Table 10 (Continued)

Area	Entropy (–) (Problems)	Evolution (+) (Resources)	Equifinality	Nursing Action
Circulation (Continued)	Transient ischemic attacks – possibly also manifested as Bell's palsy. Transient neurologic features often accompany malignant hypertension → inability to close eyes – slurred speech	Paralysis of facial muscle, speech difficulties and difficulty with swallowing is resolving – can now control both eyes 100% and speech improving	Resolved facial paralysis; normal speech and swallow reflex	3. Restrict sodium (Na+) intake per diet; watch for proteinurea, hematuria 4. Observe for proteinurea, hematuria as signs of renal damage 5. Lubricate eyes with artificial tears q1h 6. Tape eyes shut at bedtime (hs) 7. Avoid direct, harsh light in room 8. Set up communication system with pt.; be patient with her in her attempts to talk 9. Maintain pt.'s self-image in regard to palsy disfigurement 10. Prevent aspiration
	↓ Arteriosclerotic heart disease – ischemic changes (inverted T waves) in lateral precordial leads on ECG; has positive family history, also has angina pectoris. →↑ BP, has paradoxical split S_2, S_3, gallop at apex	No bruits, pulses normal, no ectopics Angina controlled with nitroglycerin sublingually	Maintain	11. Be alert for signs and symptoms of myocardial ischemia and/or impending MI (sweating, chest pain, nausea and vomiting, pallor) 12. Order ECG when there is chest pain
	↓ Multiple circulatory problems; bedrest from paralysis →↑ chance for emboli →↑ chance for skin breakdown	Many of the circulatory problems are stable at this time and complications can be prevented	Prevention of complications	13. Administer sublingual nitroglycerin for chest pain 14. Monitor vital signs carefully 15. Use TED hose while pt. is on bedrest – remove 15 min q4h

				16. Turn frequently and reposition pt. to prevent pressure sores 17. Provide meticulous and frequent skin care
Nutrition	Chronic obesity (5′4″, 183 lb) →↑ cardiac and respiratory workload →↑ energy consumption ↑ heart rate ↑ cardiac output →↑ BP	In hospital is on 1,500 calories (Am. Dietetic Assoc.) – should be able to lose weight on this	Weight loss	1. Maintain pt. on diet 2. Consult dietitian – have her see pt. 3. Encourage selection of own meals (have dietitian check)
	Difficulty in swallowing owing to Bell's palsy and Guillain-Barré syndrome →↓ intake of nutrients and fluid →↑ possibility of dehydration [4]	On clear liquid diet until patient can handle other foods – should be easy to ↓ calories	Maintenance of adequate fluid balance; prevention of aspiration pneumonia and dehydration	4. Collect intake and output data to assure adequate fluid intake 5. Prevent aspiration
	Anorexia with onset of disease – GI distress →↑ nausea and vomiting →↑ dehydration state possibility	Symptoms will ↓ weight Anorexia resolved with regression of disease	Maintain adequate nutritional state	6. Give high nutrient foods per diet to maintain nutrition, ↓ muscle atrophy rate, avoid dehydration 7. Prevent aspiration with vomiting 8. Support pt. when nauseated; reduce external stimuli 9. Administer antinausea medication p.r.n. 10. Watch for antacid →↓ gastric acidity →↓ chance of stress ulcers
Elimination	Albuminurea with onset of flu-like symptoms (from infection and/or renal damage)	Bowel function normal, no urinary sediment	Resumption of normal renal function Maintain normal bowel function Prevention of urinary retention stasis → urinary tract infection	1. Monitor temperature for urinary tract infection 2. Collect intake and output data 3. Observe for proteinuria 4. Administer stool softener while on bedrest 5. Administer milk of magnesia p.r.n.

Table 10 (Continued)

Area	Entropy (–) (Problems)	Evolution (+) (Resources)	Equifinality	Nursing Action
Sensory perception	Vague paresthesias consistent with Guillain-Barré syndrome	Paresthesias proving with resolution of paralysis	No paresthesias	1. Monitor areas and frequency of occurrence 2. Provide medication for relief of symptoms
Locomotion	Unable to move because of Guillain-Barré syndrome → ascending paralysis of somatic musculature →↑ extreme weakness Symptomatic osteoarthritis with deformity and Heberden's nodes and hip pain → makes physical therapy (PT) difficult and painful with loss of dexterity	Guillain-Barré syndrome resolving →↑ strength distally (still has proximal weakness)	Resolution of Guillain-Barré symptoms. Complete rehabilitation and resumption of normal level of functioning ↓ Arthritis pain →↑ functional activity	1. Turn frequently 2. Provide meticulous skin care 3. Provide passive range of motion exercises (q4h) 4. Provide physical therapy (q.d.) 5. Apply splints to hands and feet at h.s. 6. Administer pain medication for arthritis 7. Install trapeze so pt. can assist self with upper extremities 8. Pad handles of eating utensils thickly to facilitate manipulation
Neuroendocrine	Guillain-Barré syndrome → edema of dura around myelin sheath → degeneration of myelin sheath → paralysis of somatic musculature; is reversible	Symptoms of Guillain-Barré syndrome are resolving; respiratory involvement successfully avoided	Resumption of all normal activities without impairment	1. Be supportive 2. Give psychological support; reassure and encourage 3. Provide passive range of motion exercises 4. Apply splints to hands and feet for prevention of contractures, foot drop, muscle atrophy to excessive degree
	Bell's palsy – left-sided facial paralysis →↑ pain to jaw and behind ear → impairment in eye closure and oral retraction	Transient condition – now resolving (course usually 1 to 4 weeks)	Resolved palsy	

				5. Administer pain medications as per previous plan 6. See plans for Bell's palsy under Circulation
	Hyperglycemia (blood sugar 165 to 230 mg per 100 cc) → positive familial history for diabetes mellitus → probably influenced by obesity; possible onset of diabetes mellitus	Urines have been negative for glucose 1,500-calorie (Am. Dietetic Assoc.) diet should help control	Diet-controlled hyperglycemia	1. Double voided urines for sugar and acetone (especially since patient is on a heavy load of diuretics) 2. Check for polyurea (intake and output) 3. Monitor blood sugars 4. Maintain on diabetic diet 5. Consult dietitian 6. Provide for endocrine consultation
Reproduction	Normal	Normal postmenopausal female	Maintain	
Psychosocial needs				
Psychological	Retired Labile personality ⟷ weepy ⟷ tension headaches ⟷ insomnia ⟷ anxiety ⟷ depression ⟷ despondent [5]	Stable family life; husband, son, daughter-in-law and sister all supportive; husband retired	Psychological homeostasis ↑ Coping mechanism	1. Provide emotional support for pt.; show that she is accepted 2. Stay with pt.; reassure 3. Encourage verbalization 4. Take suicide precautions 5. Provide psychiatric consultation 6. Provide diversional activities as appropriate
Family-oriented	Normal	Normal	Maintain	1. Support family; explain disease and procedures → anxiety 2. Encourage their participation in care if appropriate

Table 10 (Continued)

Area	Entropy (–) (Problems)	Evolution (+) (Resources)	Equifinality	Nursing Action
Social	Suit pending against pt. for slander; pt. is paranoid and feels that no one in her community likes her	Has familial support with husband at home	↑ Coping mechanism	1. Allow pt. to verbalize her fears and feelings 2. Monitor visitors carefully; ↓ contact with lawyers and those involved in suit 3. Show pt. that she is accepted by the staff the way she is, without judgments being made about her
Religious	Normal	Protestant	Maintain	1. Call clergy upon pt.'s request
Nursing concerns				
Safety	Paralysis ⟷ possibility of accidents Paresthesias ⟷ possibility of accidents ↓ Swallowing reflex → possibility of aspiration or choking	Has increasing control; has gross control of upper extremities – can call for help	Prevention of accidents	1. Allow only activities pt. can safely do; provide assistance 2. Keep side rails up at all times 3. Install trapeze 4. Provide bell to call for assistance in lieu of usual buzzer, which requires more dexterity 5. Assist with meals as per plan; no hot liquids 6. Observe carefully for aspiration; have suction equipment at bedside
Instruction	Diabetic teaching	Has some knowledge of disease as sister has it; family supportive	↑ Knowledge of diabetes	1. Adhere to diet, skin care, activity, urine testing, medications

	Hypertensive teaching	Has maintained self well with medication for 6 years	Reinforce knowledge	1. Stress importance of medications; frequent B.P. checks
	Obesity teaching	By time of discharge may have a better idea of good diet and has already lost a few pounds	Good diet; weight loss	1. Stress importance of diet; exercise
	Procedures explanation	Able to comprehend instructions	↓ Anxiety because of numerous procedures	1. Explain and prepare for all procedures
Coordination of care	Numerous procedures and personnel	Able to comprehend	↓ Anxiety	1. Explain numerous personnel and their functions – how they work together to provide better care 2. Provide pt. with adequate rest periods; limit personnel when necessary 3. Provide primary nurse-advocate for this pt. so she can have one significant person to refer to 4. Plan for discharge, Public Health Nurse consultation, and contact with hometown health agencies

*Throughout, the following symbols have been used: → = causes or leads to; ↑ = increases; ↓ = decreases; and →↑ = leads to an increase.

References

1. Beeson, P., and McDermott, W. (Eds.), *Textbook of Medicine* (14th ed.). Philadelphia: W. B. Saunders, 1975.
2. Clark, M. C. Chest pain. *Heart Lung* 4:956, 1975.
3. Davies, A. G., and Dingle, H. R. Observations on cardiovascular and neuroendocrine disturbances in the Guillain-Barré syndrome. *J. Neurol. Neurosurg. Psychiatry* 35:176, 1972.
4. Gilroy, J., and Meyer, J. *Medical Neurology*. New York: Macmillan, 1975.
5. Lichtenfeld, P. Autonomic dysfunction in the Guillain-Barré syndrome. *Am. J. Med.* 50:772, 1971.

II. A Patient with Multiple Problems

Sally A. Santmyer

Mr. J. M. is a 48-year-old white man who was admitted to the hospital on March 10, 1976. (This was Mr. M.'s first hospitalization.) He was previously employed as a truck driver earning $7,000 per year and supporting seven dependents, including three children at home, aged 16, 9, and 7. On January 30, 1976, Mr. M. was dismissed from his employment and has relied on support from relatives and friends, and has used food stamps.

Three weeks prior to admission, Mr. M. had the flu with a temperature ranging between 100° to 103°F. At this time, he began drinking one quart of vodka and a six-pack of beer daily. He has a 5-year history of alcohol abuse. Five days prior to admission, Mrs. M. took Mr. M.'s alcohol away. Mr. M. became weak and confused and began seeing mice and coyotes. Mrs. M. became concerned about Mr. M.'s continual decline and brought him to the hospital. Upon admission, Mr. M. presented with symptoms of alcohol abuse, ascites, and decreased mental status. He was unable to give any history so the history was related by Mrs. M. The family has remained supportive and concerned throughout his hospitalization.

Several hours after admission, Mr. M. was noted to be somnolent and a lumbar puncture was done. Culture of the cerebrospinal fluid revealed *Cryptococcus neoformans* and an India ink test yielded positive results [2, 6]. Subsequent cultures of the urine and blood revealed the cryptococcal organism. Evidence of pulmonary cryptococcosis (by sputum culture and chest x-ray) was lacking. A regimen of amphotericin B and 5-FU was begun to combat the disseminated cryptococcosis. The 5-FU was later discontinued when a synergism study indicated antagonism between the two drugs [3].

On March 28, 1976, Mr. M.'s clinical situation was complicated by major gastrointestinal (GI) bleeding. He was transferred to the ICU; where he received iced saline lavages but they failed to stop the GI bleeding. Endoscopy revealed esophageal varices and duodenitis as possible sites of bleeding. A diagnosis of portal hypertension resulting from Laennec's cirrhosis was made. A celiac and superior mesenteric artery arteriogram was performed with the infusion of vasopressin (Pitressin) 0.2 units per minute, which halted the hemorrhage.

Mr. M.'s condition stabilized after the cessation of bleeding and whole-blood transfusions. He returned to the nursing unit on April 1.

Mr. M.'s clinical status, treatment, and nursing care have been complicated by the numerous problems he has sustained: hepatic dysfunction with encephalopathy, disseminated cryptococcal infection, particularly meningitis and the amphotericin therapy, and major GI bleeding. His encephalopathies are, at present, slowly, but progressively, decreasing, with an improvement in his clinical status. His prognosis, however, is guarded and a long hospitalization is anticipated [8, 12].

Table 11. Nursing Care Plan (Long Form) – Mr. J. M., Age 48

Area	Entropy (–) (Problems)	Evolution (+) (Resources)	Equifinality	Nursing Action
Physiological needs				
Respiration	Gross ascites compromising respirations and contributing to hypoventilation with risk of atelectasis and pneumonia	↓ Ascites and abdominal girth; paracentesis; adequate ventilation with normal arterial blood gases for area	Enhance normal ventilation Enhance ↓ abdominal girth	1. Elevate head of bed 2. Turn pt. and instruct him to cough and deep-breathe (q1h) 3. Allow pt. up in chair as tolerated and permitted by clinical condition 4. Allow progressive ambulation as above
	↑ Rales over L base	No wheezing or dullness to percussion		5. Monitor breath sounds
	History of smoking: 2 packs per day for 15 years	Has not smoked since 1973	Maintain	6. Encourage no smoking
	Cryptococcus neoformans gains access to body through respiratory tract with possible dissemination to any system, particularly brain, meninges, spinal cord [4]	No evidence of active *C. neoformans* infection in lung, scar lesions or granulomas	Maintain	7. Administer amphotericin B (Ampho B) as fungostatic agent (see Neuroendocrine)
Circulation	Atherosclerotic coronary artery disease; evidence of past lateral infarction; fixed split S_1; bruit over right femoral artery	No evidence of ongoing ischemia $S_1 = S_2$ No murmur, thrill, or heave	Promote normal sinus rhythm Prevent further ischemic attacks; minimize progression of atherosclerotic process	1. Encourage no smoking 2. Assess patient for signs of myocardial ischemia 3. Coordinate physical demands with assessment of current cardiovascular status a. When clinical situation permits, M.D. will order cardiac workup b. Gradually ↑ activity to exercise tolerance

	Tachycardia > 126 fever, withdrawal symptoms	↓ Withdrawal symptoms ↓ Fever to normal limits Pulse rate down to 70 to 90 per minute	Maintain Promote normal pulse rate	4. Administer antipyretics 5. Administer sedatives to reduce effect of withdrawal symptoms on cardiac status if clinical neuropathy permits
	↑ Cardiac rate and cardiac output, systolic and diastolic pressures with intoxicating doses of alcohol		Promote abstinence from alcohol	1. Encourage abstinence from alcohol with rehabilitation to prevent further damage to heart resulting from effects of alcohol on excitability and contractility of heart [11]
	+1 ankle edema (resulting from malnutrition and ↓ protein synthesis with consequent hypoalbuminemia [2.4 gm] and edema)		Promote good nutrition	1. Encourage abstinence from alcohol and promote adequate nutrition to correct and prevent hypoalbuminemia
	Ankle edema could be a result of congestive heart failure (CHF) as an after-effect to damaged myocardium from previously undiagnosed infarction	No clinical evidence of CHF	Maintain	1. Monitor for signs of CHF
Nutrition	↓ Food intake 3 wk prior to admission with 10-lb wt. loss Admitted with malnutrition, high protein catabolism with retention of nitrogenous waste products	Supervised food intake 20-gm protein diet composed of quality calories to prevent further malnutrition and establish Nitrogen balance	Promote nitrogen balance Prevent protein catabolism	1. Improve quality of diet within protein, water (H_2O), and Na^+ restriction 2. Gradually ↑ diet from liquids to high-calorie, bland, soft diet 3. Consult dietitian to plan meals with pt.'s favorite food within diet restrictions 4. Provide meals in pleasant atmosphere, convenient to pt.

Table 11 (Continued)

Area	Entropy (–) (Problems)	Evolution (+) (Resources)	Equifinality	Nursing Action
Nutrition (Continued)	Chronic alcoholics consume protein- and vitamin-deficient diets with clinical syndrome related to faulty nutrition			
	Blood urea nitrogen ↑ (BUN) (possible etiology is renal toxicity from amphotericin, hepatorenal syndrome, hepatic dysfunction, or blood in GI tract)	BUN ↓ (57 mg/dl)	Maintain ↓ BUN	5. Encourage pt. to eat; help if needed to aid in adequate nutrition and to ↑ strength
	Anorexia, nausea, and vomiting, etiology alcohol withdrawal or related to cryptococcal meningitis leading to ↓ food intake, ↑ protein catabolism with retention of nitrogenous waste products	↓ anorexia, nausea and vomiting with food intake ↓ withdrawal symptoms	As above	1. Achieve dietary aims when anorexia, nausea, and vomiting are present, by offering 3 to 4 small meals with supplemental feedings of eggnog and ice cream
		Concerned family	Maintain	1. Encourage abstinence from alcohol with resultant dehydration and malnutrition 2. Encourage adherence to diet; involve family in diet therapy 3. Help pt. to understand that neither nutritious diet nor added vitamins will protect his liver from further effects of alcohol
	Vitamin B deficiency (reserves of vitamin B reduced by malnutrition, diarrhea)		Provide deficiencies	1. Administer folate 1 mg by mouth daily

Elimination	Diarrhea for 3 wk prior to admission	↓ Diarrhea since admission	Promote normal bowel function	1. Monitor bowel movements as diarrhea is one side effect of neomycin
	Guaiac + stools	Site of GI tract bleeding identified; cessation of bleeding	Promote guaiac – stools	1. Test all stools and record 2. Encourage abstinence from alcohol as this was identified as cause of GI bleeding
	Bacteria generating nitrogenous products; retention of these products and those from protein catabolism with subsequent neuropathy; nephritis secondary to Ampho B or *C. neoformans* (CN growth in urine) 2+ protein, 2+ blood in urine	Receiving neomycin to reduce ammonia-forming bacteria in gut with subsequent reduction in blood ammonia results in improved neurological status; *C. neoformans* is susceptible to Ampho B [9]	Promote nitrogen balance Prevent protein catabolism Promote improved neurological function Prevent renal toxicity	1. Administer neomycin 1 gm by mouth daily 2. Be alert to nephrotoxic effects of neomycin 3. Diet (see Nutrition, GI system) 4. Administer titrating doses of neomycin 1 gm daily and Ampho B 50 mg 3 times per week 5. Dipstick urine to monitor for protein, blood spillage
	BUN (74 mg) + creatinine (Cr) (1.9 mg) (source: neomycin or Ampho B renal toxicity, blood in GI tract, or ↓ elimination of nitrogenous products)	Titration of Ampho B dose and neomycin dose Magnesium citrate to cleanse bowel of blood ↓ BUN (57 mg) + Cr (1.2) Cr not ↑ in proportion to ↑ in BUN; Cr is considered to be better monitor of renal toxicity resulting from Ampho B [7]	Promote removal of blood from bowel Maintain ↓ levels	1. Monitor BUN and Cr and alert MD to ↑ levels 2. Monitor intake and output (strictly); monitor output to detect early decrease 3. Take urine cultures as indicated for *C. Neoformans,* other bacteria, fungi 4. Administer magnesium citrate, 1 bottle daily 5. Abstinence from alcohol leading to blood in GI tract

Table 11 (Continued)

Area	Entropy (–) (Problems)	Evolution (+) (Resources)	Equifinality	Nursing Action
Elimination (Continued)				6. Diet within restrictions to prevent accumulation of nitrogenous waste products and prevent protein catabolism 7. Adequate hydration within restrictions
	Jaundiced, sclera-icteric hepatic dysfunction with hyperbilirubinemia (6.5 mg)		Promote optimal liver function	8. See GI system, above, with diet and alcohol abstinence
Gastrointestinal	Ascites – reflects complex abnormal electrolyte, H_2O, and protein metabolism that may complicate severe liver disease; results from disturbance of systemic mechanisms regulating passage of fluid and solutes across vascular and serosal membrane Hypoalbuminemia, portal hypertension, and secondary aldosteronism with Na^+ retention play role in ascites formation	↓ Ascites + abdominal girth Will usually ↓ as underlying process resolves Paracentesis – no *C. neoformans* in peritoneal fluid	Promote ↓ ascites Promote optimal liver function	1. Enforce bedrest with diuresis 2. Enforce combination of Na^+ restriction (200 to 500 mg) protein restriction (20 gm) and fluid restriction (2,000 ml) 3. Decrease ascites by means of diet and drug therapy 4. Administer aldactone 25 mg (t.i.d.) 5. Take daily weight to determine effectiveness of therapy
	3/29 Endoscopy showed esophageal varices and duodenitis; either could be site of bleeding	No tumors, ulcers, sites of bleeding in stomach	Promote optimal liver function	1. Encourage abstinence from alcohol with alcoholic rehabilitation

Laennec's cirrhosis suspected characterized by diffuse, fine scarring, loss of liver cells associated with fatty infiltration of active necrosis	Laennec's cirrhosis is basically a progressive disease but appropriate therapy and strict avoidance of alcohol may arrest the disease at most stages and permit repair and functional improvement	Promote abstinence from alcohol Enhance nutrition	1. Provide nutrition as previously discussed
Loss of liver cells because of alcohol abuse in combination with impaired nutrition leads to advancing fibrosis, which in turn contributes to the development of portal venous hypertension with resultant esophageal varices [11]	Concerned family	Maintain	1. Involve family in treatment in order to gain their support for patient
Liver scan – poor uptake of dye			
Clinical signs of cirrhosis: ↓ serum albumin and total protein, hypokalemia (3.1 mg) seen in patients with ascites and edema and secondary aldosteronism		Enhance nutrition	1. Administer potassium chloride (KCl) 15 mEq by mouth daily
Ascites – ↑ abdominal girth jaundice with hyperbilirubinemia (6.5 mg)	Clinical signs have decreased	Enhance decrease in clinical signs	1. See Nutrition, Gastrointestinal, Psychosocial
Ankle edema, hepatomegaly, ↑ weakness and fatigue, confusion and CNS dysfunction, anorexia, nausea, and vomiting			
Continued alcohol excess and poor dietary habits lead to further episodes of hepatic decompensation		Prevent further liver decomposition	

Table 11 (Continued)

Area	Entropy (–) (Problems)	Evolution (+) (Resources)	Equifinality	Nursing Action
Gastrointestinal (Continued)	Major gastrointestinal bleeding continued to hemorrhage after iced saline lavage and saline-levophed lavage ↓ Hct (40 to 29%) ↓ BP (70/0 from 106/70)	Celiac and superior mesenteric artery arteriograms for infusion of vasopressin (Pitressin) 0.2 units per ml; bleeding stopped	Maintain cessation of bleeding; prevent further bleeding	1. Maintain patency of nasogastric (NG) tube during lavage 2. Administer lavages to stop bleeding 3. Maintain integrity of vasopressin infusion with precautions 4. Do a Guaiac test on all stools for blood
		Hematocrit (HCT) ↑ to 37% postinfusion 6 units of packed erythrocytes (RBCs)	Maintain	
		BP up to normal limits	Maintain	5. Increase dietary intake gradually as elucidated under Gastrointestinal and Nutrition 6. Consider superimposed problems of ascites and possible hepatorenal syndrome; this is a *must* 7. Monitor vital signs and clinical symptoms for further evidence of bleeding 8. Alert nursing staff to possibility of further gastrointestinal bleeding because of administration of steroids with Ampho B 9. Avoid known gastrointestinal irritant 10. Establish amphogel routine

Sensory perception	↓ Effectiveness of sensory receptors as a result of hepatic encephalopathy and meningeal neuropathy			1. Attempt to maintain quiet environment 2. Maintain sense of reality – be with pt. at frequent intervals
	Visual and auditory hallucinations probably alcoholic psychosis or combination of above	↓ Withdrawal symptoms Usually alert and oriented	Enhance clear sensorium	3. Give sedatives to ensure rest and sleep if permitted by meningeal and hepatic encephalopathy 4. Keep room dimly lit at night
	↓ Mental status with confusion Visual changes and diplopia on admission (as above)			1. Explain all procedures in detail in order to alleviate fear 2. Maintain pt.'s contact with reality by presence of family member 3. Explain pt.'s symptoms to family to alleviate their anxieties 4. Monitor patient's orientation levels frequently
	Deficiency in hearing on admission (attributed to cryptococcal meningitis)	Previously intact auditory system responding to Ampho B	Promote return to normal auditory function	1. Administer Ampho B in titrating doses 2. Improve communication techniques to ensure pt.'s understanding during interim
Locomotion	Neck and trunk rigidity, cogwheel motion, almost spastic movement of extremities; unable to walk Weakness, easily fatigable	Good muscle tone ↓ weakness Now able to hold self up in chair and move from bed to chair with assistance ↓ neck stiffness ↓ tremors + asterixis	Maintain Promote normal mobility Promote self-sufficiency in activities of daily living	1. Administer passive range-of-motion exercises progressing to active 2. Maintain safety needs during weak, tremulous period

Table 11 (Continued)

Area	Entropy (−) (Problems)	Evolution (+) (Resources)	Equifinality	Nursing Action
Locomotion (Continued)	Tremulous and with asterixis (above thought to be combination of hepatic encephalopathy, withdrawal symptoms, and neuropathy from meningitis)	+ response to Ampho B		3. Attempt to maintain quiet environment, as tremors tend to diminish in quiet setting 4. Assist in activities of daily living (ADL) 5. Promote progressive activity → chair → ambulation 6. Teach pt. to ↑ his participation in his personal care gradually 7. Encourage pt. about progress 8. Involve family in care 9. Be alert to ↑ signs of entropy in locomotion
Neuroendocrine	Hepatic encephalopathy (glutamine in CSF ↑ to 20 mg/dl) in combination with cryptococcal meningitis (budding fungi-*C. neoformans* in CSF) produced following encephalopathies:	+ response to neomycin with CSF glutamine ↓ 12 mg/dl response to Ampho B; 3/26 CSF negative for *C. neoformans*	Promote absence of *C. neoformans* in CSF urine, blood	1. Assess neurological status 2. Administer Ampho B and 5-FU as ordered, increasing dose to maintenance dose (5-FU discontinued because of synergism study showing antagonism between the two drugs) 3. Be alert to side effects of Ampho B resulting from pt.'s compromised hepatic, renal, and GI systems 4. Monitor neurological signs
	Somnolence	No progressive obtundation; ↑ responsiveness	Enhance ↑ responsiveness	
	Headache	No meningismus ↓ headache	Decrease encephalopathies	
	Slow speech	Now able to talk in sentences		
	Dulled response to environment			
	Vertigo, nausea, vomiting, apathy, diplopia, and disturbed orientation			

	Absence of papilledema ↓ vertigo		5. Alert to signs of ↑ increased intracranial pressure, hydrocephalus, ↑ headaches, gait disturbances, failing intellectual function
	No evidence of space-occupying lesion from *C. neoformans*	Maintain	
	No evidence of hydrocephalus (communicating hydrocephalus documented with cryptococcal meningitis [10])	Maintain	
Pt.'s susceptibility to *C. neoformans* and its dissemination thought to be caused by lack of immunocompetence from alcoholism [7]		Promote immunocompetence	1. Encourage abstinence from alcohol leading to ↓ immunity 2. Provide adequate nutrition as previously discussed
Cryptococcal meningitis considered to be grave disorder with high mortality rate, risk of residual damage to CNS; hazards associated with therapy [1]	Improved results with Ampho B therapy when adequate doses given [1]		1. Alert pt. and family to fact that relapses occur; instruct about signs and symptoms which may occur after discharge
Side effects of Ampho B: chills, nausea, vomiting, anorexia, hypokalemia (3.1 mg), anemia, rise in serum BUN (74 mg)	Side effects can be ↓ by employing smaller doses, slowing rate of administration, by giving drug on alternate days, use of steroids or antihistamines [5] BUN elevation ↓ with titration of doses; should approach normal at conclusion of therapy [1]	Minimize side effects	1. Monitor BUN, Cr 2. Administer ↓ dosage of 50 mg Ampho B every other day over 4 to 6 hr. with 25 mg hydrocortisone 3. Administer 15 mEq KCl for hypokalemia 4. Plan diet therapy as previously described (for nausea, vomiting, anorexia) 5. Slow down Ampho B infusion if side effects occur

Table 11 (Continued)

Area	Entropy (–) (Problems)	Evolution (+) (Resources)	Equifinality	Nursing Action
Neuroendocrine (Continued)		Studies have indicated no clinical, lab evidence of permanent damage to kidneys, liver at conclusion of therapy [9] Tube agglutination and indirect fluorescent Ab test + for *C. neoformans* antibody Good prognostic sign as positive agglutin levels for *C. neoformans* develop during recovery phase when circulating antibody appears [7]		
Body integrity	Oropharynx reveals extremely poor dental hygiene with periodontal necrotizing gingivitis	Eligible for VA dental therapy	Improve oral hygiene	1. When clinical condition permits, have appointment made to dental clinic for therapy 2. Involve patient in continued plan for improving oral hygiene
		Upper dentures	Maintain	1. Recommend evaluation for proper fit to aid in nutritional intake
	Pharynx-white injected exudate – candidiasis (overall lack of immunocompetence in this pt.)	Mystatin (Mycostatin) Mouthwash	Improve general resistance Improve nutrition	1. Apply mystatin (mouthwash) 50,000 u 4 times daily 2. Refer to nursing action under Nutrition

	Ulcerative stomatitis; thought to be a result of vitamin B deficiency in debilitated patients	Folate	Correct hygiene Reduce pain Provide deficiencies	1. Administer folate 1 mg by mouth daily 2. Apply local anesthetic to reduce pain, thereby improving ability and desire to eat
Reproduction		No problems elicited by patient history or by wife	Maintain	1. Consider sequelae of hepatic encephalopathy and meningitis on sexual function
Psychosocial needs	5-year history of alcohol abuse History of alcoholism in family – father, grandfather	No previous hospitalizations for alcohol withdrawal or GI bleeding	Encourage alcoholic rehabilitation	1. Show personal interest in pt. 2. Establish rapport with pt. and see him frequently in anticipation of aiding him in alcoholic rehabilitation
	Depression over loss of job Decreased self-esteem	Previously good provider	Promote self-worth and esteem	1. Begin alcohol rehabilitation after medical crisis; such crises may help pt. to see that his alcohol problem has reached serious proportions – pt. must be willing to participate in rehabilitation or it will fail 2. Allow patient to ventilate his feelings 3. Help him to see possible solutions to his problems 4. Aid him in identifying reasons to live – to stop alcohol abuse, i.e., his family
	Wife feels pt. is more apathetic than confused	Concerned and supportive family	Maintain	
	Family financial problems	Eligible for ADC (Aid to Dependent Children) at present	Maintain support	1. Involve social worker in planning Mr. M.'s care and rehabilitation, employment, problems, current family financial problems

Table 11 (Continued)

Area	Entropy (–) (Problems)	Evolution (+) (Resources)	Equifinality	Nursing Action
Psychosocial needs (Continued)				2. Include family in planning care for Mr. M 3. Plan nursing care with time of family visits in mind 4. Watch for signs of family disruption because of alcoholism and intervene with appropriate care
Religious		Catholic, family attends Mass regularly	Maintain	1. If patient is receptive, involve priest in rehabilitation process
Cultural		Born and raised in Southwest Patient and family like living in this area	Maintain	
Nursing concerns				
Safety	Unsteady gait, weakness	Increasing strength	Prevent falls and injuries	1. Assist with activities, ambulation (see Locomotion)
	Allergy to penicillin and aspirin	Patient and family aware of allergies	Maintain	1. Avoid administration of penicillin and aspirin
Instruction	Neuropathy caused by meningitis and hepatic encephalopathy leading to intermittent periods of confusion, ↓ comprehension	Level of comprehension varies	Enhance comprehension	1. Give instructions to pt. when mental state is clear 2. Reassess instruction and reinforce 3. Promote alcoholic rehabilitation (see Psychosocial needs)

		Family interested in patient, his rehabilitation	Maintain	4. Involve family early in care, discuss possibility of relapse, their need to be aware of symptoms of relapse (cryptococcal meningitis), need to return to clinic, diet therapy
Coordination of care	Long hospitalization anticipated Several physicians directing care	Interested nursing and medical staff, student nurses	Return to optimal health	1. Be aware of each physician's plans for Mr. M.'s care 2. Coordinate pt., nursing, family, and physician's goals 3. Coordinate hospital, home care 4. Enlist aid of social agencies to provide services for pt. and family

References

1. Edward, V. E., Sutherland, J. M., and Tyrer, J. H. Cryptococcus of the central nervous system. *J. Neurol. Neurosurg. Psychiatry* 33:415, 1970.
2. Emmons, C. W., Binford, C. H., and Utz, J. P. *Medical Mycology*. Philadelphia: Lea & Febiger, 1970.
3. Fass, R. J., and Perkins, R. L. 5-Fluorocytosine in the treatment of cryptococcal and candida mycoses. *Ann. Intern. Med.* 74:535, 1971.
4. Gordonson, J., Birnbaum, W., Jacobson, G., and Sargent, E. N. Pulmonary cryptococcosis. *Radiology* 112:557, 1974.
5. Imperato, P. *The Treatment and Control of Infections in Man*. Springfield: Charles C Thomas, 1974.
6. Lewis, J. L., and Rabinovich, S. The wide spectrum of cryptococcal infections. *Am. J. Med.* 53:315, 1972.
7. Littman, M., and Walter, J. E. Cryptococcus: Current status. *Am. J. Med.* 45:922, 1968.
8. Pan American Health Organization. *International Symposium on Mycoses*. Washington, D.C.: Pan American Health Organization, 1970.
9. Sarosi, G. A., Parker, J. D., Doto, I. L., and Tosh, F. E. Amphotericin B in cryptococcal meningitis. *Ann. Intern. Med.* 71:1079, 1969.
10. Selby, R., and Lopes, N. M. Torulomas (cryptococcal granulomata) of the central nervous system. *J. Neurosurg.* 38:40, 1973.
11. Wintrobe, M. M. (Ed.). *Harrison's Principles of Internal Medicine* (7th ed.). New York: McGraw-Hill, 1974.
12. Wolstenholme, G., and Porter, R. (Eds.). *Systemic Mycoses*. Boston: Little, Brown, 1968.

III. A Victim of Trauma

Kathryn E. Smallwood

Mr. S., a 68-year-old white, single male, was admitted to the Emergency Room on February 23, 1976, after being hit by a truck. At the time of the accident, he was walking along a busy street when he was knocked to the street and sustained head and ankle injuries. For a questionable period of time, he was unconscious but upon arrival at the Emergency Room he was awake, alert, oriented as to person and time, but confused as to place, and he could not remember what had happened to him. He had a large scalp laceration in the occipital area; his eyelids were edematous, and he complained of a severe headache and pain in his left foot. He also had a large contusion of his right knee and right medial calf. His scalp laceration continued to bleed profusely in the Emergency Room despite direct pressure to the area. The physician ligated arterial bleeders with 3-0 chromic suture and after x-rays, his laceration was repaired.

After numerous x-rays, positive findings included: displaced fracture of his right medial malleolus, fracture of his left lateral malleolus with disruption of ankle joints, indicating significant ligament tearing. Skull x-rays and a sonogram were negative. Neurological findings were essentially negative, but he had brain edema and post-traumatic amnesia.

Vital signs upon admission were: BP, 120/80; pulse, 80; respiration, 24. He vomited once in the Emergency Room, his BP increased to 160/108, and then fell to 138/100; pulse, 84, then 60; respiration, 20; blood glucose, 230 mg. per 100 ml. Because glucose levels continued to be elevated, a glucose tolerance test was done on February 27, 1976. Results were – fasting value glucose: 91 mg./dl.; ½ hr., 130 mg./dl.; 1 hr., 162 mg./dl.; 2 hr., 196 mg./dl.; 3 hr., 145 mg./dl. His physician believed that the hyperglycemia was traumatically induced.

On February 24, 1976, surgery was performed: an open reduction and internal fixation of the right medial malleolus with two screws; an open reduction and internal fixation with a Rush rod of the left lateral malleolus; and repair of ankle capsule, tabofibular, and talocalcaneal ligaments. The fibulocalcaneal ligament was also sutured. Mr. S. received physical therapy after surgery and on March 3, 1976, Hexelite casts were applied.

Throughout his hospital stay, Mr. S. continued to have headaches and amnesia regarding the accident. The dizziness and vomiting subsided 2 days postinjury.

Mr. S., a retired military administrator, lives in the Northeast. He was visiting the Southwest on business and was to fly home the morning of his accident. None of his family or friends was in town. He has two brothers who live in the same city as he does and one brother who lives in Florida. All the brothers came to visit Mr. S. the day of his surgery and remained with him until his discharge on March 8, 1976. He is of Jewish (Orthodox) faith and the family is very close.

Mr. S. was in good health prior to accident. His past history reveals glaucoma for which he receives treatment with pilocarpine eye drops.

Table 12. Nursing Care Plan (Long Form) – Mr. S., Age 68

Area	Entropy (–) (Problems)	Evolution (+) (Resources)	Equifinality	Nursing Action
Physiological needs				
Respiration	No voluntary coughing to increase lung expansion since coughing increases intrathoracic pressure, which interferes with venous return from brain; increased ICP results in depression of respiratory center [1]	No trauma to respiratory system; no immediate damage to respiratory center; respirations deep and regular; negative history of pulmonary diseases and smoking	Maintain Promote oxygenation	1. Keep pt. in semi-Fowler's position 2. Keep environment dust-free 3. Monitor status; check breath sounds 4. Encourage pt. to take deep breaths
Circulation	Hemorrhage from 5-in. scalp laceration + surgery for ankle repair resulted in HCT drop from 37.2% to 28.8%, Hgb drop from 12.6 to 9.4 gm and decreased O_2 carrying capacity resulting in tissue hypoxia [4]	Arterial bleeders were ligated with 3-0 chromic sutures to prevent further hemorrhage in Emergency Room; pressure dressing applied Laceration healed well	Prevent further hemorrhage	1. Check dressing frequently for bloody drainage 2. Monitor vital signs and intravenous fluids; intake and output 3. Observe for untoward response to packed erythrocytes during infusion
		Reduced RBCs cause stimulation of erythropoietin production from kidney resulting in increased RBCs 2 units of packed erythrocytes (RBCs) given postoperatively	Increase RBCs	
	Impact to head → cerebral circulatory changes: increased hydrostatic pressure in capillaries and venules → net exchange of fluid toward tissue [5]	Cerebral blood flow autoregulates; change in diameter of the resistance vessels; blood flow remains constant during change in perfusion pressure [5]	Maintain	1. Make frequent neurological checks: assess level of consciousness, posture, and movements (motor system), including reflexes; evaluate eye movements and pupils; evaluate gross focal neurological deficit

		Alert, oriented to person and time		
		Amnesic to accident		
	Impact → displaced fracture (fx) of right medial malleolus; fracture of left lateral malleolus with disruption of ankle joints leads to edema	Right and left dorsalis pedis and posterior tibeal pulses palpated; strong, equal, regular; skin pink, warm to touch Blanch reflex in toenails normal	Prevent further injury	1. Check dorsalis pedis and posterior tibial pulses, skin temperature and color, blanch reflex of both ankles and feet frequently 2. Splint both lower extremities above and below fracture sites; pad; avoid pressure points; elevate lower extremities on pillows; apply ice; encourage pt. to move toes frequently; check sensation
	Immobilization causes venous stasis leading to clot formation	Elevation of lower extremities and ice increases venous return, decreases edema		
Nutrition	Nothing by mouth, nausea and vomiting, decreased food intake leading to catabolism of body proteins; with increased N_2 loss and negative N_2 balance Post-traumatic hyperglycemia with glucose of 230 mg/dl, 1+ glycosuria Cortisol causes increased hepatic gluconeogenesis and decreased glucose utilization by muscle and adipose tissue Catecholamine secretion causes increased glycogenolysis and lipolysis + inhibited insulin release from pancreas	Progressive diet; patient and family have negative history for diabetes mellitus	Prevent further breakdown of protein and CHO	1. Obtain past medical history re: diabetes, other nutritional diseases 2. Inform nurses on the unit that pt. is of Jewish faith; eats Kosher foods; maintain proper diet when pt. is ready to eat 3. Check urine for glucose 4. Take frequent glucose serum levels 5. Observe for signs of hyperglycemia

Table 12 (Continued)

Area	Entropy (–) (Problems)	Evolution (+) (Resources)	Equifinality	Nursing Action
Nutrition (Continued)	Glucose intolerance posttrauma from starvation; with increased glucose release from liver, decreased insulin release, decreased peripheral utilization of glucose, increased gluconeogenesis and insulin antagonism in plasma or at cellular level [5]			
Fluid and electrolyte	Some blood loss from large scalp laceration; trauma causes antidiuretic hormone (ADH) to increase H_2O retention; trauma causes adrenocorticotrophic hormone (ACTH) release; aldosterone secretion leads to Na^+ retention. Lack of correlation between serum Na^+ and Na^+ retention; mild hyponatremia may be a result of shift of Na^+ into cells but is not indicative of depletion of body Na^+ [5]	IV fluids Serum Na^+ normal	Maintain balance	1. Monitor IV fluids carefully; intake and output 2. Have blood drawn for electrolytes 3. Decrease noxious stimuli that might increase nausea; observe for Na^+ imbalance
	Increased ICP produces vomiting leading to K^+ loss; trauma results in Na^+ and H^+ movement into cell; K^+ leaves the cells [3]	K^+ metabolism not seriously affected by head injury [5] KCl added to IV; serum K^+ normal		1. Observe for K^+ imbalance

Elimination	Immobility results in decreased peristalsis, decreased food intake with decreased bulk and decreased fluids	Negative trauma to GI system; good bowel function	Maintain	1. Turn pt. frequently 2. Check bowel sounds
	H_2O retention depends on ADH action. Stimuli for release of ADH are osmotic and nonosmotic (post-trauma) factors ADH controls reabsorption of H_2O in distal convoluted tubule of nephron to maintain fluid volume + osmolarity Body trauma results in primary H_2O retention with decreased urine output, increased specific gravity, increased urine electrolytes; during period of retention, urine volume not an index of hydration and should not be used to indicate need for increased volume replacement [5]	No trauma to kidneys or bladder; no history of benign prostatic hypertrophy (BPH) or kidney disease; good urine output with normal specific gravity	Maintain	1. Monitor IV intake; monitor input and output 2. Take daily weight of pt. 3. Observe for edema; observe color and consistency of urine
Sensory perception	Trauma caused loss of consciousness at scene of accident for unknown period of time; large 5-in. laceration in occipital area; edema of eyelids; severe headache + vomiting (due to shaking of brain and/or stretching of meninges and vascular tree) [5]; post-traumatic amnesia ↓ with	Two normal sonograms. Neurological exam: indicated cerebral functioning, alert and responsive; loss of memory for accident only; cranial nerves intact Cerebellar function deferred Motor system, no atropy, weakness or tremors	Maintain; provide quiet environment	1. Reorient pt. as to what happened to him; constantly assess neurological function; avoid pain medication as it masks neurological signs 2. Avoid rough movements; provide quiet environment

Table 12 (Continued)

Area	Entropy (–) (Problems)	Evolution (+) (Resources)	Equifinality	Nursing Action
Sensory perception (Continued)	decreased sensory perception during period of accident, increased anxiety causes further increase in sensory loss History of glaucoma with increased intraocular pressure, pupils pinpoint Achilles & Plantar reflexes deferred because of fracture Trauma produces pain by following pathway: Receptors (naked nerve endings) A delta fibers — C fibers Dorsal columns — Ventrolateral columns Thalamic nuclei Reticular Activating System (arousal) — Thalamo-hypothalamic projection — Reticular Activating System	Sensory system intact to touch and pinprick Reflexes normal Uses pilocarpine eye drops to produce miosis Lower extremities splinted		3. Communicate to physician and other nurses pt.'s history of glaucoma 4. Splint fractures; elevate, apply ice; check sensation

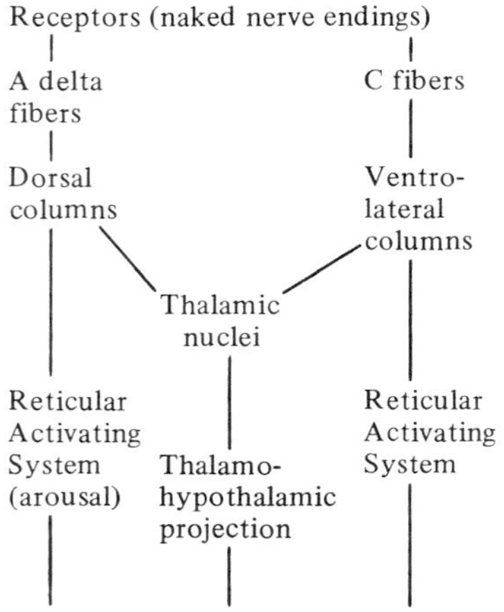

	Thalamo-cortical tract → Cortex (postcentral gyrus) → Localization of pain; Hypothalamus → Autonomic response to pain (circulation, respiration, adrenal response [1]); Thalamo-frontal projection → Cortex → "Suffering"			
Locomotion	Head injury, fracture of right and left malleolus results in immobilization causing decreased venous return, increased edema of right and left malleolar areas Head injury necessitated delayed surgery for correction with longer period of time on bedrest	Able to move upper extremities and torso	Prevent complications of bedrest	1. Turn pt. frequently, gentle movements; will not be able to turn completely on side because of splints, but prop him with pillows; avoid pressure areas; massage bony prominences and back region 2. Administer adequate fluids 3. Encourage pt. to move toes; check sensation and circulation status frequently
Neuroendocrine	Trauma causes response of all endocrine glands; direct bodily injury activates responses by (a) nerve stimulation, (b) damage to tissue cells, (c) alteration of blood volume or extracellular fluid (ECF) space; afferent nerve impulses arising from lacerated skin, subcutaneous tissue, and viscera	Hypothalamus stimulates release of vasopressin and increased BP	Prevent complications	1. Obtain medical history 2. Assess neurological function and vital signs continuously 3. Observe for hyperglycemia; monitor blood glucose 4. Decrease external stimuli, give psychological support to decrease anxiety 5. Limit IV intake so as not to increase ICP

Table 12 (Continued)

Area	Entropy (−) (Problems)	Evolution (+) (Resources)	Equifinality	Nursing Action
Neuroendocrine (Continued)	Increased intracranial pressure (ICP) increases BP	Changes in blood volume activate volume receptors in carotid arteries, kidneys, and atria and influence vasopressin secretion via osmoreceptors in carotid artery system		
	Hyperglycemia	Hypothalamus also stimulates release of ACTH leading to cortisol release which increases hepatic gluconeogenesis and decreases glucose utilization by muscle and adipose tissue. Growth hormone (GH) causes lipolysis; opposes insulin action on muscle cell while increased plasma-free amino acids inhibit muscle uptake of glucose. Adrenal medulla releases increased epinephrine and norepinephrine [3]		
	Damage to tissue cells releases K^+	Aldosterone secretion causes increased ICP which promotes Na^+ retention and K^+ excretion		

Hit by car resulting in cerebral concussion (graded set of clinical syndromes following head injury; increase in the severity of disturbance in level of consciousness; caused by mechanically induced strains affecting brain in a centripetal effect on function and structure; sequence begins at surface of brain in mild cases and goes inward to affect diencephalic mesencephalic core at most severe levels)	Neurological examination normal (no deficits noted)
Impact shears and causes strain, leading to coma, confusion, and amnesia	Resolves to normal consciousness
Increased ICP may be a result of indentation of cranium at point of impact; effect of acceleration and deceleration more important with peak of ICP occurring when brain, continuing to travel in one direction, strikes rebounding calvarium, with sharp increase in ICP and development of pressure gradients at time of impact; resultant deformation and flow of brain tissue from high to low pressure regions; loss of	

Table 12 (Continued)

Area	Entropy (–) (Problems)	Evolution (+) (Resources)	Equifinality	Nursing Action
Neuroendocrine (Continued)	consciousness and changes in BP are almost result of physical changes in brain and not cerebral blood flow [5]			
Reproduction	Trauma results in increased adrenal androgens, decreased libido [1]; hospitalization	Mature adult; understands hospitalization necessary	Maintain	1. Explore and allow expression of feelings; answer questions pt. may have
Psychosocial needs				
Psychological	Injury causes sudden disruptive situation; fear and anxiety with post-trauma amnesia causes stress and crisis. Pt. does not live in town; family support not present; no friends here; increased anxiety stimulates neuroendocrine system.	Crisis can be growth-promoting; independent, he wanted to wait to call family when he could talk with them Allowed staff to call hotel to make sure luggage was in safe place and to cancel plane reservation	Promote communication Decrease anxiety	1. Reorient pt. to what happened to him and what is being done for him and why 2. Notify family and friends when pt. is ready 3. Respect independence and individual worth 4. Allow him to express his fears and anxieties 5. Identify coping mechanisms 6. Communicate to staff on the unit Emergency Room assessment of psychological needs
Social	No friends to call; family in Northeast	Interacted well with staff; accepted need for dependence upon them	Maintain	1. Introduce self and others to pt. 2. Allow pt. to call family as soon as he is ready

		Retired military administrator, unknown business now; active person; had insurance-Medicare; 2 brothers in Mass. and 1 brother in Florida		
Cultural	Away from home Crisis situation	Jewish faith; close family ties; independent; likes to make own decisions re family and business	Maintain	1. Respect individual worth 2. Communicate to nurses on unit that pt. eats kosher foods; notify dietary as soon as able to take p.o. foods
Religious	Unfamiliar to surroundings	Jewish faith – Orthodox; follows tradition	Maintain	1. Ask pt. if he wishes rabbi notified; communicate with staff
Nursing concerns				
Safety	Post-trauma amnesia; increased ICP; limited activity; lower extremity splints	Alert, oriented; understands limitations	Provide safe environment	1. Side rails up; protect sites of injury; keep laceration dressing clean, dry 2. Reorient pt. at intervals
Instruction	Confusion because of unfamiliar surroundings, and post-traumatic amnesia with increased anxiety and decreased cognition	Alert, intelligent	Provide information Decrease anxiety	1. Reorient pt.; give simple explanations; alert staff to pt.'s progress
Coordination of care	The number of hospital personnel add to confusion and anxiety of patient Does not live in town; not familiar with physician and hospital	Previous hospitalization	Provide therapeutic environment	1. Introduce pt. to staff as they provide care 2. Explain what will be done and why 3. Communicate to staff on unit: history of pt., care received in Emergency Room; emphasize psychosocial needs

References

1. Beland, L. *Clinical Nursing: Pathophysiological and Psychosocial Approaches.* New York: Macmillan, 1970.
2. Ommaya, A. K. *Head Injury Mechanisms.* Bethesda: National Institute of Neurological Diseases and Stroke-NIH, 1973.
3. Shoemaker, W. C., and Walker, W. F. *Fluid-Electrolyte Therapy in Acute Illness.* Chicago: Year Book, 1970.
4. Sodeman, W. A., and Sodeman, W. A., Jr. *Pathologic Physiology: Mechanisms of Disease.* Philadelphia: W. B. Saunders, 1974.
5. Vinkin, P. J., and Bruyn, G. W. (Eds.). *Handbook of Clinical Nephrology: Injuries of the Brain and Skull, Part I.* New York: American Elsevier, 1975.

IV. A Victim of Cerebrovascular Accident

Linda L. Brommer Bustamante

Mr. B., a 56-year-old male, had experienced fairly good health until the onset of this illness. During the third week in January, he suddenly collapsed at work and lost consciousness. Co-workers had noticed some asymmetry of his face and speech difficulty prior to this incident.

On admission to the hospital he was obtunded, but he could respond appropriately to simple commands. An angiogram revealed total occlusion of the right internal carotid artery with left subclavian steal syndrome. On the basis of his neurological workup, it was decided that Mr. B. had had a cerebral vascular accident (CVA) involving both the brain stem and pons.

The patient's physical condition stabilized but he responded poorly to most rehabilitative measures. It was believed that his response was a result of depression rather than the CVA, but this was difficult to determine. A psychiatric consultation recommended electrotherapy, a recommendation not acted on by the medical doctors.

There has been a gradual but definite improvement in Mr. B. He has become more responsive and verbal and is starting to assume some measures to help himself. The prognosis is still not known. One neurologist thought he could become independent in his activities of daily living, but this will depend upon his mental status.

Table 13. Nursing Care Plan (Long Form) – Mr. B., Age 56

Area	Entropy (–) (Problems)	Evolution (+) (Resources)	Equifinality	Nursing Action
Physiological needs				
Respiration	Right lower lobe (RLL) pneumonia Infiltration inhibits exchange of gas between atmosphere and alveoli; can result in hypoxemia from ↑ PCO_2 with less alveolar space for O_2; ↓ respiratory exchange with CO_2 retention can cause diffuse cerebral edema	Treatment initiated early; pt. responded well to treatment; arterial blood gases (ABGs) showed ↑ PO_2 after O_2 administration ↑ PO_2 increases O_2 supply to the brain	Facilitate resolution of the pneumonia	1. Promote adequate rest 2. Observe vital signs closely for early signs of increased infection 3. Note changes in color, amount, and consistency of sputum; note type, depth, and rhythm of respirations with any changes [5] 4. Administer antibiotic to maintain adequate serum level; watch for any complications of drug administration or of pneumonia, i.e., stiff neck
	Rarely coughs, or deep-breathes; ↓ in ability to move secretions mechanically up airway; secretion good media for bacterial growth, further complicates the pneumonia Ineffective coughing ↑ intrathoracic and intracranial pressure; both should be avoided in this patient	When pt. does cough, he has a deep, strong cough, preceded by a deep breath; this aids in removal of secretion and improves aeration of lung	Facilitate removal of secretions	1. Try to elicit spontaneous cough by stroking neck [2] 2. Do percussion followed by postural drainage within limits of cardiac status 3. Ascultate lungs to determine individual needs for drainage 4. Encourage high intake of fluids 5. Check for pleuritic pain which may hinder deep respirations and coughing

Table 13 (Continued)

Area	Entropy (–) (Problems)	Evolution (+) (Resources)	Equifinality	Nursing Action
Respiration (Continued)			Maintain patent airway	1. Suction as needed; use as little suction as necessary to remove secretions to reduce trauma [2] 2. Use sterile technique to prevent introduction of pathogens into respiratory tract [2] 3. Watch for changes in patient's color both in bed and when up; give O_2 when indicated
Circulation	Swelling of right wrist as a result of venous hydrostatic pressure caused by interference of blood flow through veins with ↑ filtration of fluid	No injury to wrist; swelling is reduced with elevation; this ↓ venous hydrostatic pressure; range of motion (ROM) ↑ interstitial pressure through the massaging action of muscles	Facilitate venous return	1. Support paretic arm with sling when pt. is up to reduce pain and edema 2. Elevate right extremity when pt. is in bed 3. Do not permit right arm to hang in dependent position 4. Watch for increased swelling 5. Apply ROM to right hand and arm 4 times a day [6]
	History of hypercoagulability of venous blood. May be aggravated by ↓ movement that causes ↓ return of blood to heart from lack of compression of muscles against veins	No evidence of thrombophlebitis; ROM given regularly to aid the "muscle pump"	Maintain venous return	1. Turn pt. regularly with avoidance of positions that result in excessive pressure, especially in calf of legs [3] 2. Use properly fitting elastic stockings for lower extremities 3. Have each shift of nurses remove stocking and inspect pt.'s legs for irritation and constriction; keep stockings smooth [8]

			4. Elevate pt.'s legs or use footstool when sitting him up 5. Check for edema of feet 6. Teach patient, when he is able, to press against footboard and other exercises to improve venous return
Ulcer on left ankle, slow to heal; ↓ nutrition and ↓ PO_2 inhibit tissue repair	Ulcer is not infected or open; ulcer on nonparalyzed leg; movement will ↑ circulation; tube-feeding supplies protein needed for tissue maintenance	Facilitate healing of ulcer	1. Keep ulcerated area clean with gentle washing; inspect regularly for early signs of infection or increase in size 2. Handle left ankle gently; prevent any trauma to this area 3. Keep pressure off by use of footboard and proper positioning
Recent MI; occurred prior to admission; myocardial necrosis present resulting from ↓ O_2 needed to support metabolic functions; this patient showed ↓ cardiac output aggravated by blood viscosity from dehydration, his immobility, and by hypoxemia	No chest pain; PVCs controlled with medication; no increase of myocardial damage after admission; enzymes ↓ at gradual rate; no apparent decompensation	Maintain adequate cardiac function Reduce further cardiac injury	1. Check vital signs for any changes; check pulse for rate, rhythm, and irregularities 2. Observe closely for chest pain, restlessness, or anxiety 3. Treat pain promptly with medication 4. Check peripheral pulses for indications of inadequate cardiac function [2] 5. Note patient's color; give O_2 6. Watch for signs of hypotension, especially a drop in BP or urinary output, less than 30 cc per hr.; BP must be maintained to preserve systemic circulation [7]

Table 13 (Continued)

Area	Entropy (–) (Problems)	Evolution (+) (Resources)	Equifinality	Nursing Action
Circulation (Continued)				7. Avoid sudden physical effort 8. Do passive exercises of all joints; initiate more active exercises when ordered 9. Watch for early signs of CHF such as dyspnea, cough, or rhonchi
	Reddened areas over bony prominences; hyperemia is result of cell destruction and hemorrhage resulting from prolonged pressure and lack of O_2 and nutrients for tissue needs	No decubitus formation; reddened areas improved with measures to ↑ circulation	Maintain good skin tone without breakdown	1. Careful and regular observation of skin for signs of irritation 2. Begin circulation-stimulation massage on bony prominences [2] 3. Support the entire body to prevent injury when transferring pt. 4. Do not keep pt. up in wheel chair for long period of time; help pt. to reposition self while up 5. Use a firm mattress for better distribution of weight
Nutrition	Pt. eats poorly; is losing weight; adequate nutrition needed for maintaining metabolism, body temperature, and synthesis of new tissue; ↓ intake causes electrolyte imbalance	NG tube-feeding started and tolerated well; family willing to supplement tube feedings with pt.'s favorite foods	Maintain adequate nutrition; prevent weight loss	1. Pt. should be watched for signs of electrolyte imbalance when he is not eating; after tube feedings are instituted, pt. should be fed at regular times

Pt. takes inadequate fluids resulting in dehydration; this ↓ body's heat regulation mechanism, ↓ transportation of nutrients, and O_2 to cells and waste products away from cells	Fluid replacement through tube relieved the dehydration	Facilitate hydration, without overloading pt.	1. Give oral hygiene three times a day; keep nares clean and well lubricated to reduce irritation from NG tube 2. Check skin turgor and mucous membranes for signs of dehydration; keep accurate record of intake and output; weigh pt. to determine fluid retention
Chokes at times	No evidence of aspiration pneumonia Able to cough deeply No paresis of facial muscles for chewing	Facilitate intake; maintain patent airway	1. Give specific instructions on feeding the pt. to family and personnel; suction machine should be kept at bedside at all times; watch for signs of respiratory distress
Nausea and vomiting may result from midbrain infarct [1]; this ↑ fluid loss, which ↑ the dehydration; it ↑ electrolyte loss, especially Na^+ and Cl^-; as food intake ↓, protein catabolism ↑, both may aggravate the diabetes; vomiting ↑ cardiac stress	Vomiting is controlled with medication; electrolytes are within normal limits after initiation of tube feedings	Facilitate adequate intake; reduce vomiting	1. Aspirate before each tube feeding to determine amount in stomach to prevent overfeeding, which may result in regurgitation and vomiting [4]; pt. should have head elevated to 45° for feeding; after this, pt. should gently be turned to his side to reduce possibility of his aspirating the feeding 2. Let pt. rest after each feeding; check for proper placement of tube before feeding to determine possible dislodgement; give antiemetics as needed

Table 13 (Continued)

Area	Entropy (–) (Problems)	Evolution (+) (Resources)	Equifinality	Nursing Action
Elimination	Incontinent of urine; bladder sensation and control may be ↓; contributing to problem are dehydration, immobility, depression, and difficulty with communication	Indwelling Foley patent; no evidence of bladder infection; pt. becoming more responsive, may soon be able to indicate his needs	Maintain Foley patency; reduce trauma to bladder	1. Give at least 3,000 cc per day if tolerated by cardiac condition; try to maintain acid urine by diet [8]; prevent overdistention of bladder by careful observation of output, and signs of restlessness; observe urine closely for cloudiness or sediment – possible signs of infection 2. Tape catheter to pt.'s abdomen to prevent penile-scrotal fistula [2]; give meatal care every 8 hours
	Incontinent of stool; loss of sensory and motor function needed for evacuation; adding to problem are ↓ in food and fluid intake, ↓ physical activity and difficulty in expressing needs	No history of constipation; good response to bowel routine, with minimum to straining which could ↑ intrathoracic and intracranial pressure	Facilitate good bowel routine	1. Perform bowel routine at same time each day, following pt.'s prestroke bowel habits; avoid bedpan if possible for better evacuation and less stress
	Skin irritation on buttocks resulting from the ammonia present in urine along with other acid and alkali components	Skin intact without signs of open areas	Maintain skin integrity	1. Keep skin scrupulously clean; use absorbent pads to aid in removal of moisture; note any new or increased areas of irritation; ointment to protect skin may be used if irritation persists

Sensory perception	Dysarthric mumble; damage in the basal part of pons can affect right pyramidal tract with paralysis of part of the tongue, soft palate, and some superficial muscles of face	Speech gradually improving; pt. can be understood	Facilitate improvement in speech	1. Speak slowly; use easily understandable words; let pt. repeat words after personnel; try to anticipate pt.'s needs to prevent excessive frustration; do not overstimulate pt. 2. Stand in front of pt., since there may be loss of visual field [2]; speech therapist should evaluate pt.
	Does not verbalize at most times	Has ability to communicate verbally and nonverbally	Facilitate some type of communication	3. Try to understand pt.'s nonverbal communication; same personnel should work with pt. to know pt.'s needs better
	Very little interest in environment	Has understanding of spoken word; shows more alertness at times	Improve pt.'s awareness of environment	4. Try to keep pt. in social world; take advantage of pt.'s periods of increased awareness; learn about pt.'s background and use this in communication with him [8] 5. Help pt. with his personal hygiene and appearance
	Eyes reddened; pt. rarely blinks	No infection noted; good vision	Maintain good vision	6. Keep pt.'s eyes clean; inspect for signs of infection or irritation; apply moisturizing solution to eyes every shift to prevent dryness
	Unilateral deafness may occur with pons infarct [1]	Pt. had good hearing before stroke Hears when spoken to in a normal tone of voice	Maintain adequate hearing	7. Speak in normal tone of voice; don't shout; try to ascertain pt.'s understanding of what was said; try to determine if pt. has hearing impairment; speak to pt. from unaffected side

Table 13 (Continued)

Area	Entropy (–) (Problems)	Evolution (+) (Resources)	Equifinality	Nursing Action
	Difficulty with temperature sensation may occur with brain stem infarct [1]; this is from damage of the spinal tract of trigeminal nerve		Facilitate pt. comfort and safety	8. Keep pt. comfortable based on environmental conditions; remember that pt. is not aware of too hot or cold objects; teach pt. safety precautions when he is more alert and responsive
Locomotion	Right-sided paresis; lesions in the basal portion of the pons can include the pyramidal tract causing an upper motor neuron type of paralysis	Good strength in left hand; uses left hand in purposeful movements; physical therapy (PT) daily	Maintain strength of left side of body	1. Provide good support for upper right extremity to prevent subluxation of shoulder [8]; use footboard to prevent footdrop; prevent external rotation of hip with trochanter roll; provide wrist and finger extensor splint for the paretic hand; passive ROM t.i.d.; do muscle strengthening exercises when pt. is ready; gradually increase pt.'s tolerance to sitting, which is impaired by weakness and change in sense of balance [1]; follow through PT program on ward; support pt.'s right leg when in bed to prevent it from falling downward and forward, which results in dislocation

	Flaccid paralysis generally gives way to spasticity in brain-stem injuries [7]; spasticity will often result in deformity caused by the ↑ strength of the flexor and adductor muscles; deformities result from body's attempt to ↓ pain [2]	Pt. has no contractures of joints; PT daily; nurses do ROM several times daily; ROM stimulates circulation, helps to reestablish neuromuscular pathways, prevents muscular contractures and joint stiffening	Maintain good joint mobility	2. Position pt. on nonparetic side and supine for most of day to ↓ pain and trauma; position pt. so there is no strain on any joint; pain sensation may be lost on the affected side and the pt. may not be able to recognize his uncomfortableness [7]; pt. must always be in good body alignment to prevent contractures 3. Turn pt. frequently, at least every 2 hr 4. Put trapeze on bed when pt. shows ability to help self 5. Note increased resistance of joints; extra attention should be given to these joints
Neuroendocrine	Borderline diabetic; could be aggravated by ↓ food intake and protein catabolism resulting from tissue damage and immobility	Diabetes well controlled after pt. placed on tube-feeding; pt. received about 2,000 calories per day; diet meets pt.'s protein and electrolyte needs – both protein and K^+ needed for insulin production	Maintain diabetic control	1. Record urine sugar and acetone; report any glycosuria; give correct diet; report inability of pt. to tolerate diet
	Massive CVA of brain stem involving midbrain and pons, resulting from thrombus There is ischemia of the brain tissue supplied by affected vessel and edema and congestion in surrounding area	Pt.'s condition stabilized after 2 days without evidence of increased infarction	Maintain stable state	1. Watch pt. closely for signs of increased infarction, and especially cerebral edema shown in reduced awareness; note any rise in temperature, pulse rate, or respiratory rate – as these can be early signs of a fatal CVA

Table 13 (Continued)

Area	Entropy (–) (Problems)	Evolution (+) (Resources)	Equifinality	Nursing Action
Reproduction	Problems with sexual activity cannot be ascertained at this time	Unknown at this time	Recognize pt.'s needs when indicated	1. Be alert for pt.'s concern or questions about sexual functioning 2. Obtain outside counseling if necessary when pt. expresses a need for it
Psychosocial needs				
Psychological	Sudden loss of productivity; increased depression while in hospital; past history of mild depression Depression can be a result of pt.'s being placed in a dependent situation; he initially had difficulty with communication; he had loss of body function, with threat to self-concept	At times pt. seems more alert; seen by psychiatrist; responds to family at some times	Increase periods of alertness; reduce depression	1. Stimulate pt. when he seems more alert; observe pt.'s response to antidepressive medication; be honest in dealing with pt.; accept pt. with his feelings; be aware of psychiatrist's thoughts concerning pt.; be consistent and follow through, utilizing his suggestions; when pt. is more alert, include pt. in planning his care; be realistic in explaining to pt. about his condition; talk with family about depression associated with disability [8]; be supportive of family
Family orientation	Had become increasingly less responsive to family	Family able to visit often; they show a willingness to help pt.; seem realistic in their understanding of pt.'s condition and prognosis	Maintain family's understanding. Help them with their feelings.	1. Give family positive, realistic support; family needs opportunity to talk [4]; accept their feelings; involve family in future plans involving pt.; let them assist in the care of the pt. if they want to do this

Social	Has been a "loner" in past with few friends; has no visitors except family	Family is supportive	Facilitate pt.'s socialization; maintain family support	1. Personnel and family should continue to demonstrate interest in pt.; be alert to pt.'s interest in some activity; learn about pt.'s interests from family and try to utilize this information; when caring for pt. talk to pt. explaining what is being done and why; do not ignore pt., although he does not respond verbally
Religious	Does not attend church; family not aware of pt.'s religious preferences; no needs expressed by pt.	Pt. has increased ability to express his needs	Meet pt.'s spiritual needs as he communicates them	1. Be alert to the expression of a need for spiritual help; try to ascertain what is important to the pt. to anticipate his religious needs [2]
Nursing concerns Safety	Pulls at NG tube and Foley catheter	No evidence of bladder infection; no bleeding from nose	Prevent injury or trauma to self	1. Apply mitts to pt.'s hands to restrict his pulling on tubes 2. Observe for hematuria or signs of bladder infection; medicate for restlessness if indicated 3. ROM to hands and wrists twice a shift if mitts are used; check hands for edema
	Had pulled self over foot of bed and fallen	No injury from fall; posey jacket adequately restrains pt. in bed	Maintain pt. safety	4. Use posey jacket to prevent pt. injury both in bed and while sitting up; closely supervise pt.; check posey often to make sure it is not too tight so that it may compromise respirations; watch for skin irritation under posey straps

Table 13 (Continued)

Area	Entropy (–) (Problems)	Evolution (+) (Resources)	Equifinality	Nursing Action
Safety (Continued)	At times, pt. strikes out at others when care is given	Alert at times; understands what is told him	Facilitate personnel safety	5. Give good explanation of what personnel are doing before care is given; treat pt. as an adult; use two people for better control of pt.; be alert to pt.'s needs; minimize pain in caring for pt.
Instruction	Seems too depressed at times to want to learn	Shows increased alertness at times; understands what is told him	Facilitate pt.'s understanding and learning	1. Always tell pt. what is being done and why, using simple terms; when pt. is more alert, try to get feedback about his level of understanding; let pt. make decisions about his care when he is able
Coordination of care	Does not want to be disturbed for care, either by nursing or other disciplines	Generally accepts care in a passive manner	Provide care needed by pt. with a minimum amount of stress or threat	1. Do not confront pt. with daily change; maintain a fairly constant schedule; try to understand the pt. and his needs [2]; coordinate activities which consider the pt.'s needs resulting in setting of priorities; same people should care for pt. with good continuity of care; provide a therapeutic relationship by trying to understand pt.'s needs and feelings

References

1. Beeson, P., and McDermott, W. (Eds.). *Textbook of Medicine* (14th ed.). Philadelphia: W. B. Saunders, 1975.
2. Beland, I., and Passos, J. *Clinical Nursing: Pathophysiological and Psychosocial Approaches* (3d ed.). New York: Macmillan, 1975.
3. Brunner, L., and Suddarth, D. *Textbook of Medical-Surgical Nursing* (3d ed.). Philadelphia: J. B. Lippincott, 1975.
4. Carini, E., and Owens, G. *Neurological and Neurosurgical Nursing* (5th ed.). St. Louis: C. V. Mosby, 1974.
5. Kintzel, K. *Advanced Concepts in Clinical Nursing* (2d ed.). Philadelphia: J. B. Lippincott, 1975.
6. Luckman, J., and Sorensen, K. *Medical-Surgical Approach to Nursing.* Philadelphia: W. B. Saunders, 1974.
7. Wintrobe, M. (Ed.). *Harrison's Principles of Internal Medicine* (7th ed.). New York: McGraw-Hill, 1974.
8. Zankel, H. *Stroke Rehabilitation.* Springfield, Ill.: Charles C Thomas, 1971.

V. A Patient with Multiple Sclerosis

Ellen Kval Isaak

Mrs. S. M., a 55-year-old mother of three grown children, was born and raised in New York but later moved west with her husband, who is a physician. She experienced no serious illness, trauma, or disability prior to 1960, when she had a hysterectomy. Following the surgery, she experienced episodes of tingling and numbness all over her body, followed by weakness in her lower extremities. By 1965, her diagnosis of multiple sclerosis had definitely been confirmed, as she exhibited progressive weakness, and increased gamma globulin was found in the cerebral spinal fluid [6, 8]. By 1972, she was confined to a wheelchair. On April 1, 1976, she was admitted for a general checkup because of gastrointestinal disturbances and increasing generalized weakness in her upper extremities. Mrs. S. M. was discharged on April 6, 1976, following her tests.

Table 14. Nursing Care Plan (Long Form) – Mrs. S. M., Age 55

Area	Entropy (–) (Problems)	Evolution (+) (Resources)	Equifinality	Nursing Action
Physiological needs				
Respiration	Moderate obstructive ventilatory defect (↓ vital capacity) probably resulting from neuromuscular problems; upper thoracic lesion interferes with intercostal breathing	Pt. does not smoke; up in chair so gravity aids deep breathing by relieving pressure on diaphragm	Enhance ventilation	1. Monitor vital signs; encourage pt. to cough and deep-breathe slowly 2. Change pt.'s positions often
	Upper respiratory infection (URI) frequent cause of death in multiple sclerosis (MS) [4, 7]	No URI	Maintain	3. Protect from URI, smoke, dust, airborne irritants [2]
Circulation	Wolff-Parkinson-White syndrome (accelerated conduction syndrome [5], type B, involving left bundle branch; atria activates ventricles prematurely, via accessory route and normal pathway; can cause tachycardia and life-threatening arrhythmias [5]	Pt. alert, able to report episodes; propranolol (Inderol) 10 mg q. 8 hr (↑ as tolerated) prolongs refractiveness of the atrioventricular (AV) node and ↓ or abolishes window created by discrepant refractory periods of the two pathways	Prevent tachycardia	1. Observe pt.; monitor vital signs; administer medications; avoid precipitating factors of fatigue, stress, overexertion
	Propranolol can cause symptomatic bradycardia; propranolol is a β-blocking agent which inhibits adrenergic stimulation	BP averages 120/80; pulse averages 90 to 100; normal electrolytes; hemoglobulin, and hematocrit		2. ROM exercises; skin and foot care; frequent position changes; ↑ legs at times to enhance venous return; possible support hose
	General muscle weakness; paraplegia; ↓ venous return, ↑ venous stasis, pooling in dependent parts, feet edematous	Pt. attuned to position changes and requesting assistance	Enhance circulation to lower extremities	

Nutrition	Intestinal complaints over years from ↓ mobility and peristalsis; upper thoracic lesion could interfere with peristalsis	5′ 2½″, wt. 110 lb; swallowing unimpaired; Festal, 1 tablet with meals, provides more digestive enzymes to relieve GI discomfort from excess intestinal gas; pt. knowledgeable re: nutrition; desires to remain as independent as possible	Maintain nutritional status	1. Encourage wt. maintenance; observe for signs of difficult swallowing (often occurs in late stages); encourage bulk in diet; monitor calcium intake
	Slight intention tremor; weakness in upper extremities; paraplegic		Maintain independence	2. Assist only as needed, e.g., to open small packets; accept occasional spills; allow pt. to eat slowly; suggest self-help devices for home use (Arthritis Foundation is good resource)
Elimination Bowel	Paraplegia; generalized weakness; lack of sphincter tone and control; patients with neurogenic disease prone to development of fecal impactions	Not incontinent; negative for occult blood, for ova, and parasites; Dialose, 1 capsule h.s., has water-retaining and lubricating properties to provide fecal softening effect; psyllium hydrophilic mucilloid (Metamucil), 1 tsp. in A.M. provides smoothing effect and bland nonirritating bulk to promote natural elimination; glycerine suppository; the irritant action of demulcent promotes bowel evacuation; Medicone suppository, a local anesthesia, controls muscle	Establish program of regularity	1. Periodically test stool for occult blood; administer medications; ↑ fluid intake; ↑ bulk in diet; monitor bowel action; insert glycerine suppository after breakfast and assist to bathroom one half hour later; instruct pt. to bear down, contract abdominal muscles and apply pressure to abdomen with hands to assist defecation 2. Digitally remove fecal material as necessary

Table 14 (Continued)

Area	Entropy (−) (Problems)	Evolution (+) (Resources)	Equifinality	Nursing Action
Elimination				
Bowel (Continued)		spasm and with emollients provides assistance with bowel evacuation		
Urinary	Repeated, recurrent urinary tract infection (UTI) over years	Urine cultures negative	Maintain	1. Ensure good perineal hygiene 2. Ensure adequate fluids to flush urinary tract
	Moderate-to-severe urethral stenosis; detrusor dysfunction of hypotonic nature (probably from upper lumbar lesion)	Urethral dilatations over years kept pt. relatively free of UTI	Maintain	3. Monitor voiding schedule; observe for urgency, frequency, incontinence
	Generalized weakness; paraplegia; tendency for residual urine; and renal calculi from high urinary excretion of calcium [9]	Current urinary output adequate; being up in chair aids output via gravity; pt. drinks cranberry juice with meals in attempt to acidify urine	Maintain	4. Instruct pt. to aid urine flow by coughing, contracting abdominal muscles, manually compressing lower abdominal wall; frequent position changes; ↑ fluid intake to 3 to 5 liters daily to prevent salts from precipitating out in the urine; monitor urinary pH and specific gravity
	Urinary tract infection common cause of death in multiple sclerosis	pH of urine 6; specific gravity 1.005		
Sensory perception				
Auditory	Normal		Maintain	
Olfactory	Normal		Maintain	
Visual	Some nystagmus, some oculomotor involvement; sensitive to bright lights	Uses sun and reading glasses	Maintain	1. Avoid glaring lights; protect and keep glasses in reach; observe for further visual impairment of optic nerve; use verbal communication

Touch	Loss of vibration sense in lower extremities; also some position sense lost; upper extremities have weakness and intermittent involvement; paresthesia; hence, pt. more susceptible to pressure areas	Rest/exercise program Pt. consciously inspects pressure areas for signs of heat and redness	Maintain skin integrity Enhance pt. participation	1. Observe pt. for pressure areas; protect from heat, cold, pressure, irritants; provide good skin care; encourage pt. in activities of daily living (ADL)
Locomotion	Paraplegia, with muscle-wasting from disuse; some weakness of upper extremities from cervical lesions; upper thoracic lesions; trunk unstable; confined to wheelchair since 1972; sometimes pleasantly resists cooperation with physical therapy	Up in chair as tolerated Assists in moving self in bed Instructs staff on position of comfort; physical therapy	Enhance any physical movement Enhance	1. ROM exercises; place objects in reach; employ safety precautions; encourage activity to tolerance; observe for fatigue; encourage pt. participation in scheduling rest-exercise programs with PT; encourage verbalization
Neuroendocrine	Multiple sclerosis of 14-yr duration; lesions throughout CNS; cerebellar symptoms, marked ↓ of manual dexterity, intention tremor Generalized spastic weakness; paraplegia; paresthesia, especially in legs; loss of vibration sense (evidence of lesion of posterior columns; spasticity and ↑ deep tendon reflexes primarily a result of inhibitory influences on gamma motor neurons [3]	Pt. inspects pressure areas for heat and redness Diazepam (Valium), 2.5 mg 2 to 4 times daily, provides relief from skeletal muscle spasms and spasticity from upper motor neuron disorders; pt. determined to remain as active as possible; pt. knowledgeable re: medical facts of multiple sclerosis	Minimize flexor spasm at knees and hips; maintain skin integrity; prevent and treat muscle spasticity; prevent muscle contractures and loss of muscle power from disuse	1. Sleep mostly prone 2. Change pt.'s position at least q2h prone, to lateral, to supine; skin care, with attention to pressure areas; dry, wrinkle-free bed 3. Foam mattress over firm base, or, if possible, alternate pressure mattress; possible sheepskin

Table 14 (Continued)

Area	Entropy (–) (Problems)	Evolution (+) (Resources)	Equifinality	Nursing Action
Neuroendocrine (Continued)	Bedsores and complications, common cause of death in multiple sclerosis, with severe spasticity accompanying paralysis; feet reddened; diazepam has CNS depressant effect; side effects that mimic multiple sclerosis include fatigue, ataxia, confusion, constipation, depression, diplopia, dysarthria, headache, incontinence, changes in libido, nausea, changes in salivation, tremor, urine retention, vertigo, and blurred vision; slightly ↑ alkaline phosphatase most likely caused by ↓ muscular activity and calcium metabolism in bone (paraplegia) [1]	General skin condition is good; no skin breakdown; no contractures; pt. cooperative Normal thyroid function, cholesterol level, triglycerides, lipid profile, and SMA-12, except for alkaline phosphatase	Prevent joint contractures; enhance independence Prevent equinovarus deformities of feet Maintain	4. Avoid skin trauma (heat, cold, pressure, friction of sliding); encourage best use of remaining physical power; encourage pt. in ADL, active and passive ROM, and muscle-stretching daily; avoid muscle fatigue by stopping just short of fatigue; encourage verbalization, pt. participation; suggest self-help devices while observing pt., and assist as necessary; administer medications; supply footboard; possibly have pt. wear shoes at night if problems arise
Reproduction	Hysterectomy in 1960; right breast mastectomy in 1973 (cancer with axillary node involvement)	No further evidence of cancer	Maintain	1. Encourage pt. to ventilate feelings, concerns
	Left breast shows slight thickening at 0200 position; unable to repeat mammogram because of positioning	Not believed significant		
		↑ alkaline phosphatase of 95 mg per 100 cc (high normal, 85) believed a result of paraplegia		

Psychosocial needs				
Psychological	Ego-threatening disability; prognosis: uncertain life expectancy; quality of life affected	Middle-aged mother; wife; college graduate; high intelligence; strong determination; varied outside interests; pleasant and cooperative; shows acceptance of multiple sclerosis; knowledgeable about multiple sclerosis; no financial stresses; family independent	Enhance	1. Accept pt.; reinforce positive aspects; encourage ventilation; encourage pt. in her living with disability and making the most of assets; allow pt. to participate fully in her care/health plan; enhance pt.'s independence; avoid being too helpful; overgenerous offers of help, if unchecked by pt., may undermine sense of independence, lower morale, and foster dependency wishes 2. Observe for signs of euphoria, depression, intellectual deterioration, as cranial nerves may be involved
Social	Frequent visitors interfere with rest/exercise program	Concerned husband and 3 grown children; visitors important for psychosocial interactions	Maintain Balance	1. Include family 2. Enlist aid of pt. in scheduling social activity around PT, tests, and rest; monitor fatigue levels
Cultural/Religious		Jewish (conservative)	Maintain	1. Consider culture and beliefs
Nursing concerns				
Safety	Multiple sclerosis of 14 yr; spastic paraplegia; generalized muscular weakness	Highly intelligent; knowledgeable about multiple sclerosis	Expand; maintain safe environment; maintain reasonable standard of physical fitness	1. Siderails up; necessary objects within easy reach; secure safely in chair; carefully select roommate; protect from fatigue, physical or emotional stress, infection, trauma, and ↑ temperatures, as these are possible causes for exacerbations of multiple sclerosis [2]

Table 14 (Continued)

Area	Entropy (–) (Problems)	Evolution (+) (Resources)	Equifinality	Nursing Action
Instruction		Highly intelligent	Enhance and reinforce knowledge	1. Explain therapy, tests; answer questions as they arise
Coordination of care	Multiple physicians' tests, visitors, therapy, activity; cannot tolerate busy, stressful schedule (believed one cause of exacerbations of multiple sclerosis)	Knows limits; cooperative	Therapeutic environment	1. Have pt. exercise moderation in all activities; no long waits in x-ray, etc.; coordinate visits of all involved with care 2. Suggest Multiple Sclerosis Society or Arthritis Foundation for self-help aids [8]

References

1. Adams, C. W. M. *Research on Multiple Sclerosis.* Springfield, Ill.: Charles C Thomas, 1972.
2. Brunner, L. S., and Suddarth, D. S. *Textbook of Medical Surgical Nursing* (3d ed.). Philadelphia: J. B. Lippincott, 1975.
3. Clark, R. G. *Manter and Gatz's Essentials of Clinical Neuroanatomy and Neurophysiology* (5th ed.). Philadelphia: F. A. Davis, 1975.
4. Elliott, F. A. *Clinical Neurology* (2d ed.). Philadelphia: W. B. Saunders, 1971.
5. Gallagher, J. J., Svenson, R. H., Sealy, W. C., and Wallace, A. G. The Wolff-Parkinson-White syndrome and the preexcitation dysrhythmias. *Med. Clin. North Am.* 60(1):101, 1976.
6. Krupp, M., and Chatton, M. J. *Current Medical Diagnosis and Treatment.* Los Altos, Calif.: Lange Medical Publications, 1975.
7. McAlpine, D., Lunsden, C. E., and Acheson, E. D. *Multiple Sclerosis: A Reappraisal* (2d ed.). Baltimore: Williams & Wilkins, 1972.
8. *National Advisory Commission on Multiple Sclerosis,* (Vols. 1, 2) U. S. Department of Health, Education and Welfare. DHEW Pub. No. 74-534. 1974.
9. Poser, C. M. Recent advances in multiple sclerosis. *Med. Clin. North Am.* 56(6):1343, 1972.

General Systems Theory Nursing Care Plans: Short Forms

11

I. Short Form Used in the Emergency Room

Kathryn E. Smallwood

A plan of care should begin the moment a patient enters the health care system. Many emergency rooms serve outpatients – for example, those who receive blood transfusions and intravenous medication over an indefinite period of time. A written plan of care for these patients, as well as for those who are acutely ill, would prove most helpful to those giving them care. Time is a critical factor in the emergency room, and a care plan should be quick, flexible, and easy to understand. The general systems theory care plan has these characteristics. Patient assessment can be quickly recorded and the plan of care determined. The plan allows for rapid changes in nursing care and evaluation of care.

The following plan was used in an emergency room for Mrs. C. F., a 66-year-old patient who had an asthmatic attack and who was later admitted to the hospital. It could be adapted for use by nurses on a medical unit, thus providing better continuity of care.

Table 15. Nursing Care Plan (Short Form) – Mrs. C. F., Age 66

Area	Entropy (–) (Problems)	Evolution (+) (Resources)	Equifinality	Nursing Action
Physiological needs				
Respiration	Asthma with bilateral inspiratory-expiratory wheezing; hypoxia	O_2, IV fluids; aminophylline 500 mg IV; SoluCortef 250 mg IV	Provide adequate oxygenation; relieve bronchospasms and congestion	Maintain pt. in semi-Fowler's or Fowler's position; administer O_2 per cannula; check breath sounds; monitor medication and IV fluids; check arterial blood gases
Circulation	Hypoxia; with decreased O_2 to coronary vessels; myocardial ischemia; questionable history of myocardial infarction	O_2 per cannula; bedrest; takes digitoxin (Crystodigin)	Provide adequate O_2; decrease workload of heart	Monitor vital signs with cardiac monitor; observe for arrhythmias; explain purposes of equipment; ask pt. about pain; keep nitroglycerine tablets at bedside; check intake and output; observe for symptoms of congestive heart failure
Nutrition	Allergy to tomatoes, possibly other foods; obesity	Avoids allergy food; has decreased caloric intake; lost 10 lb	Maintain	Review diet, discuss allergy foods; correct misconceptions
Elimination	History of diverticulitis	Takes psyllium hydrophilic mucilloid (Metamucil), Mylanta; no recurrence in 4 yr; aminophylline increases urine output; no history of renal disorder	Maintain	Maintain adequate hydration; exercise will be problem because of cardiac function; laxative may be needed; determine usual time for defecation; monitor input and output and daily weight
Sensory perception	Near-sighted Increased anxiety	Wears corrective lenses 4-yr history of asthma	Maintain Decrease anxiety	Inquire as to date of last eye exam; explain to pt. what is being done

Locomotion	Bedrest	Range of motion (ROM) not limited	Promote ROM	Encourage pt. to move extremities while in bed; turn pt. often; check peripheral pulses
Neuroendocrine	Stimulation of all endocrine glands	Stimulation needed to meet demands	Prevent complications	Monitor all body systems and effect of medications; allow pt. to verbalize fears and anxieties
Reproduction		No children Hysterectomy 20 yrs ago	Maintain	Obtain thorough history
Psychosocial needs				
Psychological	Illness-anxiety Afraid she was dying prior to Emergency Room admission; lives alone	Mr. D., a close friend and neighbor, helped her; has insight: able to verbalize feelings; admitted she does not like to live alone, especially when she has asthmatic attacks	Maintain; promote expression of feelings	Let Mrs. F. verbalize how she felt during asthmatic attack and ways she dealt with past attacks; call Mr. D. when Mrs. F. admitted to hospital or discharged home; keep him as well as pt. informed of her progress
Social		Has many friends; family lives in Ohio but talks with them often	Maintain	Call Mr. D; ask Mrs. F. if she wants family called; place phone within reach
Cultural		Well-educated black; retired school teacher and principal; enjoys reading and follows current events	Maintain	Give her time to talk about her past; she enjoys this
Religious		Protestant, attends church regularly	Maintain	Ask if she would like minister or chaplain to be notified
Nursing concerns				
Safety	Allergies to tomatoes and and dust; toxic effects of medication; bedrest	Pt avoids dusty areas; room provided away from "dusty" environment; pt. avoids tomatoes	Provide therapeutic environment	Maintain environment as dust-free as possible; observe effects of medication; notify dietary re food allergies

Table 15 (Continued)

Area	Entropy (–) (Problems)	Evolution (+) (Resources)	Equifinality	Nursing Action
Instruction	Increased anxiety	Intelligent, M.A. in Education; eager to learn and take care of herself	Increase knowledge	Learn what she does know and let her verbalize; assess readiness to learn and review medications and allergies with her; have dietitian visit to review diet
Coordination of care	Numerous hospital personnel	Same private physician for 4 yr Previous hospitalization	Increase knowledge	Explain to her various procedures and tests to be done and generally who is to do them; encourage her to ask questions; obtain assistance from various disciplines by increasing communications

II. A Patient with Multiple Entropies

Peggy Sue MacMacken

Mr. C. M., a 51-year-old white male, was admitted to the hospital on April 5, 1976, with severe persistent right upper quadrant abdominal pain radiating to his back. The pain started the evening prior to admission, and was associated with nausea, vomiting, and some diarrhea.

Mr. C. M. admitted to drinking about fifteen shots of whiskey each day; this practice had been going on for years. Approximately a week previous to this admission, he began having right upper quadrant discomfort. He attributed this to peptic ulcer disease, which he has had for approximately the last 13 years. He denied any tarry stools or rectal bleeding with this illness, but stated he had had bleeding from the ulcers on occasions in the past.

Mr. C. M. stated he has had diabetes for approximately 18 years and has been taking phenformin (DBI) 50 mg. q.d. He denied following any specific diet, or even requiring any insulin. He has also had a history of hypertension, for which he has taken Regroton daily. His blood pressure has been around 140/80.

His family history is significant in that his father and a sister were diabetic. There is also a history of hypertension in the family.

The patient smokes three packs of cigarettes per day, and has done so for years. He states that approximately 4 to 5 years ago he became slightly jaundiced from "liver trouble" but does not know if this was attributable to heavy drinking or not. He has had no recent jaundice.

Assessment by his physician on admission resulted in the following diagnoses: (1) acute pancreatitis (serum amylase 5,000 units), (2) alcoholic, (3) peptic ulcer by history, (4) hypertension (controlled), and (5) diabetes mellitus.

Table 16. Nursing Care Plan (Short Form) – Mr. C. M., Age 51

Area	Entropy (–) (Problems)	Evolution (+) (Resources)	Equifinality	Nursing Action
Physiological needs				
Respiration	Pt. smokes 3 packs of cigarettes per day and has for many years; some rhonchi in right lung base posteriorly	Pt. denies shortness of breath; no temperature elevation; lungs generally clear to percussion and auscultation	Maintain adequate respiratory exchange	Discourage smoking; instruct patient as to reasons Instruct pt. to turn, cough, and deep-breathe at least q.2h. while on bed rest
Circulation	History of hypertension	Regroton daily seems to control hypertension; BP 140/80 Heart not enlarged. No murmurs or arrhythmias; strong femoral and pedal pulses No edema of extremities	Maintain normal BP Prevent circulatory shock	Monitor BP closely; observe for signs of circulatory shock
	During acute attack of pancreatitis, plasma may be lost into abdominal cavity, which diminishes blood volume; acute pancreatitis causes increased vascular permeability, resulting in potential peripheral vascular collapse and shock [5]			
Nutrition	Drinks 15 shots of whiskey per day	Appears well nourished (6′1½″, 196 lb), takes oral vitamin supplements occasionally at home; receiving vitamins IV while NPO	Provide proper nutrients	Monitor weight; begin discharge planning in terms of proper diet; enlist assistance of dietitian

	History of peptic ulcers	No recent symptoms related to ulcers	Maintain	Continue use of antacids p.r.n. when NG suction is discontinued
	Patient is NPO and on continuous NG suction	Removal of stomach acid raises pH of duodenal contents, thus decreasing pancreatic secretion through the secretin mechanism [1]	Decrease production of enzymes; remove acid secretion from stomach; prevent ileus	Measure gastric contents Observe and record color and consistency of drainage; observe NG tube for patency
Elimination	Has had tarry stools in the past from ulcer disease; stools from acute pancreatitis patient usually bulky, pale, and foul-smelling (fat content varies 50 to 90%, normal 20%) [6]	No recent GI bleeding; stools of normal color and consistency; fat content analysis not done	Maintain	Observe character of stools
Sensory perception	Severe abdominal pain (from edema and distention of pancreatic capsule, and peritoneal irritation)	Meperidine (Demerol) relieves pain with minimal effect on Oddi's sphincter; effective in relieving pt.'s pain	Relieve pain; allay apprehension	Medicate p.r.n. and give tranquilizers as ordered
	Morphine sulfate has more potent stimulating action on Oddi's sphincter and is therefore contraindicated [4]	Frequent turning relieves pressure and aids in preventing pulmonary emboli and vascular complications		Change position frequently
Neuroendocrine	History of diabetes for past 18 years; blood glucose on admission 246 mg/dl; follows no special diet	Takes phenformin (DBI) t.d. 50 mg q.d.	Control diabetes	Monitor blood glucose levels; clinitest as indicated
		Does clinitest b.i.d.; shows no spillage	Prevent hyperglycemia	Begin planning for discharge teaching re: diet, follow-up, etc.

Table 16 (Continued)

Area	Entropy (–) (Problems)	Evolution (+) (Resources)	Equifinality	Nursing Action
Neuroendocrine (Continued)	Serum amylase and lipase increase caused by interference in normal outflow of these enzymes from acinar cells and through ductal system of pancreas into duodenum	Antispasmodic and anticholinergic drugs reduce gastric and pancreatic secretions Bedrest decreases body metabolism thereby reducing enzyme secretion; pt. receiving probantheline (Pro-Banthine) and Donnatal	Minimize pancreatic secretions	Bedrest as ordered; planned rest periods when allowed up
	Amylase 5,000 u on admission, 170 u on discharge; lipase 2.8 u on admission, 2.1 u on discharge			Give medications as ordered
	Loss of calcium is related to the presence of fat necrosis and formation of calcium soaps in tissues [3]; patient's serum Ca^{++} 8.1 mg/dl		Maintain normal calcium level; prevent tetany	Monitor blood levels of serum calcium; observe carefully for signs of tetany
	Electrolyte losses occur as result of continuous NG suction, severe diaphoresis, emesis, being in a fasting state	Patient receiving IV replacement (Na^+, K^+, Cl^-); receiving trimethobenzamide (Tigan) p.r.n. nausea; has had no emesis since admission; lab reports show electrolytes within normal range	Maintain proper balance of fluid and electrolytes	Keep accurate intake and output record Monitor electrolytes

Psychosocial needs				
Psychological	Patient is middle-aged alcoholic; alcohol causes spasm of Oddi's sphincter; obstruction of pancreatic duct	Appears to be of average intelligence	Provide psychological support; decrease and ultimately eliminate alcoholic intake	Be alert to pt.'s mental and emotional changes from alcoholic withdrawal
	Pt. seems to have some underlying psychological problems; admits drinking to some, denies it to others; appears rigid in thinking, easily angered; has difficulty developing trusting relationships with others			Attempt to establish good rapport with the patient; explore his feelings re A.A.; include his family (if indicated); possible psychiatric consultation
Family-oriented	Avoids talking about his family	Wife and two teen-aged children live with him; apparently in good health	Elicit support of family members to help patient cope with his illness	Observe interactions with family for clues for intervention
Social	No apparent problems	Average socialization; attends group functions, etc.	Maintain	
Religious		Family Catholic; pt. professes no preference in faith		Respect pt.'s right to his own beliefs
Nursing concerns				
Safety	Problems regarding safety appear to be related to teaching patient about his illnesses and maintenance	Possesses ability to understand illnesses and implications for care	Educate patient to prevent progression and recurrence	(See Instruction)

Table 16 (Continued)

Area	Entropy (−) (Problems)	Evolution (+) (Resources)	Equifinality	Nursing Action
Instruction	Alcohol and coffee increase pancreatic secretions; spicy foods and heavy meals are strong gastric stimulants [2]	Has apparently "controlled" his diabetes and peptic ulcer disease for many years	Educate to prevent progression and recurrence of existing illnesses	Instruct in importance of diet; avoid alcohol, spicy foods, coffee, heavy meals, eating when nervous or tense, etc.
				Emphasize importance of keeping follow-up appointments, taking prescribed medications, etc.
				Instruct in small, frequent feedings (patient discharged on 1,000 calorie low-fat diet)
Coordination of care		No significant problems in hospital setting		Suggest that social worker or VNA follow-up home visit might facilitate home care; discharge coordinator might assist in discharge planning

References

1. Beeson, P. B., and McDermott, D. (Eds.). *Textbook of Medicine* (14th ed.). Philadelphia: W. B. Saunders, 1975.
2. Carey, L. C. (Ed.). *The Pancreas.* St. Louis: C. V. Mosby, 1973.
3. Dreiling, D. A., Janowitz, H. D., and Perrier, C. V. *Pancreatic Inflammatory Disease – A Physiologic Approach.* New York: Hoeber Medical Division, Harper & Row, 1964.
4. Elliott, D. W. Acute pancreatitis. *Emergency Medicine* 6(4):24, 1974.
5. Gambill, E. E. *Pancreatitis.* St. Louis: C. V. Mosby, 1973.
6. White, T. T. *Pancreatitis.* Baltimore: Williams & Wilkins, 1966.

III. A Patient with Cardiovascular Disease

Roberta Ann Palmer

Mr. M. A., a 50-year-old Mexican-American, was admitted to the hospital on April 14, 1976, with a diagnosis of cerebrovascular disease.

Previously in good health, Mr. M. A. had complaints of hearing a "humming" sound in his ears for 5 days prior to admission. On April 14, 1976, he awoke with numbness and weakness in his left arm. He also has vertigo, visual disturbances, and an episode of dyspnea on exertion without chest pain or referred pain. He is found to have a high blood sugar and may be prediabetic. He has a positive familial history for cardiovascular disease and hypertension.

His workup includes a lumbar puncture, cerebral angiography, 2-hour postprandial glucose, cardiology, and ophthalmology consultations. Possibilities are (1) CVA, (2) intracranial aneurism, (3) cardiac arrhythmias, or (4) slow myocardial infarction. As some form of new vascular accident is obvious, the best diagnosis at this time seems to be cerebrovascular insufficiency secondary to vascular disease, possibly arteriosclerosis.

Mr. M. A. has been married for 30 years and has four children. He is an electronics technician currently employed and lives in the city.

Table 17. Nursing Care Plan (Short Form) – Mr. M. A., Age 50

Area	Entropy (–) (Problems)	Evolution (+) (Resources)	Equifinality	Nursing Action
Physiologic needs				
Respiration	Episode of severe dyspnea on exertion Apr. 4, 1976; has smoked 1½ packs per day for 30 yr	Never been dyspneic on exertion before; no nausea or vomiting, palpations, or chest or referred pain with episode	Avoid dyspneic episodes; find and treat cause	Observe for dyspnea with exertion Observe respiratory pattern Assist patient; avoid strenuous activity until cause found Instruct patient to inform nurse if short of breath Have O_2 available in room Discourage smoking
Circulation	"Humming" in ears; weakness and numbness of left arm; decreased sensation in left hand; vertigo; right carotid bruit; visual disturbances; right blurred; left cataract; familial history cardiovascular and hypertensive disease	Pupils equal and reactive; ECG normal; not hypertensive; no angina; no diplopia; no gait changes; all reflexes normal; bilateral symmetry; no recent trauma	Prevention of accidents; catch impending CVA	Watch frequently for neurological signs Assist with ambulation; use safety precautions Check VS and BP and all pulses frequently Have patient report all changes in sensation Explain all procedures; lumbar puncture, cerebral angiography pending
Nutrition	Normal	Normal	Maintain	Allow pt. to choose own diet
Elimination	Normal	Normal	Maintain	Assist to bathroom because of vertigo
Sensory perception	Numbness of right hand; visual disturbances; cataract on left; sight blurred on right; history of eye surgery at age 9 for photophobia	Blurriness clearing; probably from incorrect lenses per ophthalmology consultation	Prevention of accidents	Allow no hot liquids Observe for extension of numb areas Have pt. report all visual changes

Locomotion	Vertigo	Has not fallen – only feels dizzy; transient sensation	Prevent accidents	Assist with ambulation Provide walker or side rails Bed rails up, bed close to bathroom
Neuroendocrine	Elevated blood sugar; may be prediabetic Neurological signs as under Circulation	No familial history of diabetes	Confirm or rule out diabetes and regulate/control	Check urine for spilled sugar Administer check 2 hr postprandial Diabetic teaching if indicated
Reproduction	Normal	Normal		
Psychological needs				
Psychological	Worried about symptoms and questionable diagnosis	Has familial support	Decrease anxiety	Support patient Supply information; answer questions/explain procedures Allow pt. to verbalize
Family-oriented	Normal	Normal	Decrease family's anxiety	Support family Answer questions; explain procedures
Social	Normal	Normal	Maintain	Allow open visiting hours Give patient pass Apr. 18
Nursing concerns				
Safety	Vertigo; decreased sensation	Has not fallen; is oriented; will ask for help	Prevention of accidents	Assist with ambulation and care Avoid hot liquids or sharp objects in room Keep side rails up at HS Provide room close to bathroom
Instruction	May be prediabetic; high blood sugar	No familial history	Increase knowledge of disease	Provide diabetic teaching if indicated
Coordination of care	Numerous procedures and personnel	Pt. is able to comprehend	Decreased anxiety	Explain all procedures and functions of personnel Provide primary reference personnel for pt. and family

IV. A Patient on Dialysis

Deborah L. Oakes

Mrs. R. S., age 49, entered the hospital to have an arteriovenous shunt placed in her right arm so that she can receive dialysis due to her hypertension, which has not been controlled with medication. Mrs. R. S.'s health is further compromised by her obesity, diabetes mellitus, and arteriosclerosis. To guide her care, a nursing care plan, short form, was devised.

Table 18. Nursing Care Plan (Short Form) – Mrs. R. S., Age 49

Area	Entropy (–) (Problems)	Evolution (+) (Resources)	Equifinality	Nursing Action
Physiological needs				
Respiration	Rales in lower lobes; history of pulmonary effusion	No orthopnea; normal easy respirations	Maintain normal respiratory patterns	Check lungs for adventitious sounds; check for fluid retention
Circulation	Atherosclerosis; arteriosclerosis; poor circulation to extremities; minimal activity	Dialysis regulates BP; decrease weight by 50 lb; no edema present; all dry weight	Maximize circulation; minimize progression of atherosclerosis	Encourage use of polyunsaturated fats; monitor BP closely; encourage activity
Nutrition	High-protein catabolism – azotemia; moderately obese; retains K^+ and fluids; Na retention	40-gm protein diet; restriction of fluids and K^+ and Na; moderate carbohydrates and fats for energy	Decrease protein catabolism; maintain near normal blood glucose level; maintain normal nutrition	Reinforce diet; encourage limitation of fluids; consult dietitian
Sensory perception	Occasional confusion	Glasses with bifocals; sees well with glasses; alert and oriented most of the time; dialysis		Reinforce necessity of good foot care; encourage safe environment; check orientation
Locomotion	Obese; weakness; little activity; more prone to blood clots	Able to move about; lower weight by 50 lb; weakness is lessening; enjoys gardening	Increase activity; prevent thrombophlebitis	Encourage exercise and increased activity; encourage garden work
Hygiene	Shunt in right arm; pt. is right-handed; limits ability to shower and wash hair; diabetics are more prone to infections; shunt and wound from CVP sites for entrance of bacteria	Sees beautician q. wk.; husband helps with shower; plastic glove covers shunt during bathing; antibacterial ointment to CVP site	Maintain good hygiene; prevent infections	Reinforce need for good hygiene; more prone to infection Apply sterile dressings over shunt and CVP site

Table 18 (Continued)

Area	Entropy (–) (Problems)	Evolution (+) (Resources)	Equifinality	Nursing Action
Hygiene (Continued)	Excretion of protein catabolites via skin pores – causes itching – excessive scratching → open sores – back and legs	Diphenhydramine (Benedryl) relieves itching to some degree	Relieve itching as much as possible	Encourage use of lotions
Neuroendocrine	Diabetes mellitus neuropathy – feet and fingers; dialysis – hormone and electrolyte imbalance	Insulin U-100, 15 u; self-injections; no reactions, stable glucose (200 mg/dl); good foot care; well educated	Maintain near-normal glucose; regulate electrolyte balance	Check glucose level; reinforce foot care; check for sensation changes; check serum electrolyte levels
Reproduction	Starting menopause	Accepts changes in menstrual cycle; no abnormal depression or mood swings; no "hot flashes"; 2 children	Maintain acceptance of changing reproductive abilities	Encourage verbalization of feelings
Psychosocial needs				
Psychological	Tries to conceal concerns about illness; great anxiety about finding a kidney donor	High intelligence; family support; sister is being considered for possible compatibility as donor	Acceptance of illness; acceptance of reality that a donor may not be available for some time	Encourage verbalization of feelings; let pt. progress at own pace; stress positiveness; encourage independence
Family-oriented	11-year-old son – changes in schoolwork since mother's illness; pt.'s 2 brothers are both borderline diabetics and are therefore not possible donors	Husband is supporting and accepting of wife's condition; 17-year-old daughter helps with household chores, drives pt. to the dialysis unit; son's teachers are understanding and willing to help	Maintain family unit; acceptance of mother's illness by son	Discuss son's progress in school with pt. and husband; possible conferences with teacher; help pt. understand why son is behaving the way he is – encourage verbalization of feelings; possible psychological consultation; include family in teaching, discussions, and planning of care; encourage normalcy of daily life patterns

Social	Leave of absence from much loved work; weakness → ↓ activities	Many friends and former students visit frequently; strong desire to return to work	Return to somewhat normal life style	Discuss possible part-time working position; encourage social activities and verbalization of feelings; recommend Diabetes Association
Religious		Normal for patient; is Presbyterian – no strong religious commitments	Maintain	
Nursing concerns				
Safety	Neuropathy Increased susceptibility to infections. Weakness → ↓ activity → more susceptible to thrombosis; visual disturbances	Good understanding of diabetic complications; daughter drives car for pt.; maintains good foot care	Prevent accidents; prevent infections; prevent thrombus formation	Check for progressive changes; encourage activity and exercise; reinforce prevention of infections; immediate treatment for infections and stress; assess home situation for safety
Instruction	Occasionally confused as a result of azotemia	High intelligence; good understanding of illness; is at learning stage with illness; desires to know more about illness	Adequate understanding of diabetes mellitus, its complications, and treatment	Progress at pt.'s own pace for learning; check for learning cues; instruct and reinforce understanding about: diet, foot care, eye changes, and diabetes mellitus complications, needs due to dialysis, pathology of diabetes mellitus
Coordination of care	Hostility and confusion toward physician	Will be seen by renal team from now on; all needed services are at the Medical Center, e.g., dietitian, physicians, possible psychologist for son	Acceptance of new doctors	Help pt. understand reasons for the change in services when a diabetic begins dialysis; coordinate all care

Student Views 12

I. One View of General Systems Theory

Judith Twitchell

The general systems theory is realistic and applicable. It is easily understood and makes the nurse feel she is part of a team instead of an isolated entity trying to be "all things to all people." It is realistic in that the responsibility of patient care is shared. It is broadening because it affords the opportunity of working with other health disciplines and learning what their skills can contribute toward achieving our goal – patient health (or death with dignity).

The tool used covers all aspects of the patient and returns individuality to the patient, instead of referring to him or her as "Room 634, Bed 1," or "the Choley in Room 634." Individuality is vital, as the patient is now a major contributing factor in his own care instead of being placed in the role of the "receiver." In other words, the patient's needs are now established primarily by the patient. The information is collected in one spot for immediate referral. With the material all in one place, anyone on the health team can use it, update it, correct it, suggest approaches, and thus instigate interdisciplinary communication. Although the nurse is the initial contact with the tool and the patient, the nurse is no longer burdened with the total responsibility for the patient's care. That responsibility is now shared. This tool can act as a true motivational factor for the nurse. It stimulates professionalism through the need for research in order to increase the value of her input to the total care of the patient. It also requires the nurse to assess the patient physically and psychologically, thus considering the *total view*. Finally, it stimulates the need for improvement in the problem-solving process and the assessment of nursing needs.

Although the tool is extensive and comprehensive, the needed information can be obtained from the patient interview, chart research, and input from several resources. To complete the tool requires team effort; it can easily be updated at nursing shift changes or through discussions at any time throughout the day. This open system allows a "multiplicity of variables that permits a continuous exchange in an orderly process with outcome not totally predictable due to the number of variables.... The stress of the interactions between those involved in the *total care* of the patient serves a purpose..." by lessening the number of variables and making the outcome somewhat more predictable. Constructive "... criticism is the result of concern," and the concern is for the patient, resulting in nursing action based on "reason not ritual."*

Feedback in this system comes from several souces: other health team members, the patient, the family of the patient, and from the nurse herself.

All components of the tool are precise and concise. The needed information is simple and well defined. The form does not require a great deal of time; it can be filled out in a short period (10 to 20 minutes) once the assessment has been thought through. It can be utilized for short-term or long-term patients.

The one problem with the tool, however, is that there is no area for listing the patient's medical history, and therefore no comparison with the present illness or observations of integration of past behavior can be made. It also does not allow for presentations of already-tried approaches to a problem noted under Nursing Action. It seems to be a *now* care plan. Nor is there an accomplished area, unless this could be noted via a date in red ink or some other form of communicating the fact.

In summary, this theory and tool are true assets in the total care of a patient. The nurse can mentally utilize the plan on every patient with whom she comes in contact.

Also, this tool can be used by a prospective teacher of nursing most effectively. A student in a clinical setting would find it most helpful in arranging the care to be given to the patient as well as supplying the reasons behind giving that care. The Entropy and Evolution sections remind the student that although there are problems present, there are positive factors working for that patient. It could easily be used for feedback to the student as to what she or he had overlooked or had observed properly. If completed prior to giving care, it could enhance the student's observations and make them more thorough. At the time of charting, the tool could be used to provide an immediate reminder for improvement of information relayed through accurate charting.

The truly outstanding factor in the use of this tool is its availability and the ease with which it can be read. Any literate person can read the presented data and obtain information which would be helpful for a therapeutic relationship.

II. General Systems Theory: Positive and Negative Aspects

Roberta Ann Palmer

Positive Aspects

At first glance, nurses probably find that the most impressive aspect of this theory for care planning is the fact that it promotes consideration of the entire patient. This can be both positive and negative – the negative aspect will be discussed later. A positive aspect of the theory is that it corresponds exactly

*Quotations from A. Putt, unpublished material, 1976.

with the basic nursing philosophy of involving the entire patient in his care and healing process. This philosophy is drilled into all nurses from the time they enter their basic educational programs and, indeed, is one of the major reasons many nurses reject medicine in favor of nursing as a profession. This has implications for the utilization of the theory because nurses tend to use only what they see is related. What use is a theory for nursing if it is so far removed from nursing philosophy that nurses cannot identify with it? In answer, the theory will be rejected and lie dormant and unused.

The positive aspect of individualization is related to this same concept. General systems theory allows for each patient to be considered from the viewpoint of his own unique condition and set of surrounding circumstances. This again is in keeping with basic nursing philosophy and hence promotes utilization. Failure to consider or depend on individualization is one of the largest factors in the rejection by nurses of standardized care plans. Considering the individuality of patients and approaching each individual's therapy from his own unique position and lifespace are the essence of nursing.

Another positive feature of the general systems theory is that, in addition to its consideration of the entire individual, it is quite comprehensive. The recent trend toward specialization in nursing does not absolve nurses from their mandate to assess and provide scientific and complete nursing care. On the contrary, nurses need to continue to develop new and better ways of delivering their unique brand of health care. The general systems theory allows nurses to develop and rationalize their care openly and for the record.

Two factors, (1) the increasing specialization of nurses and (2) the extremely rapid pace of technological and scientific advancements, have made it increasingly more difficult for nurses to keep abreast with that which they feel is professionally demanded of them – that is, to know everything about everything! The general systems theory can function as an educational tool in this respect by pointing out areas to the particular nurse involved in that patient's care of which the nurse really does not have more than a basic knowledge. This implies several things: (1) additional reading and study in that area by the nurse, (2) inservice implications for the inservice director, and (3) multidisciplinary or intradisciplinary consultations. Therefore, the general systems theory is viewed as being quite conducive to opening lines of communication between and within health professions.

The general systems theory for nursing is quite conducive to joint nurse-patient care planning as well. This again relates to the utilization of the tool and the fact that this theory is complementary to nursing philosophy. By emphasizing positive aspects (as seen in Evolution) in conjunction with the problems (Entropy), the patient can be guided to a more objective view of his disease process. This has tremendous implications for rehabilitation. The goals (Equifinality) can be arrived at jointly by the nurse and patient and add realistic objectivity to the entire plan.

One large area in care planning where many approaches fail is in the consideration of sociocultural aspects and differences. General systems theory provides for this; the entropy may not necessarily be a problem in one culture whereas in another it may be devastating. The same holds true for evolution and equifinality. General systems theory allows for these sociocultural differences should the nurse be perceptive enough to pick them up – and hence her nursing action would be directed toward the reestablishment of homeostasis in the patient as it is perceived by that patient.

Overall, the general systems theory for care planning is not so complex or time-consuming that it would not be used – the fate which befalls the best of care plans if they are too cumbersome. As a result, general systems theory is workable and utilitarian and would help to solve the communications gap within and between health care professions and as a result contributes considerably to consistency in patient care.

Negative Aspects

One of the criticisms of general systems theory of care planning is that some necessary categories are omitted. For example, the overt communication problem (while an imaginative person could fit this in under different categories) in some cases deserves emphasis. This would help to underscore the importance of that problem.

On the other hand, in some cases the plan tends to be repetitious, making it cumbersome; this in turn decreases its usefulness. For example, a cerebrovascular accident may fit in under the headings Circulation or Neuroendocrine. To avoid being redundant, it is often difficult to decide what category is the best in any given instance.

The long form of the general systems theory care plan is indeed too cumbersome for floor use while the short form often fails to demonstrate interactions between different disease processes in a multiproblem patient.

There also seems to be no place for multidisciplinary intervention. For example, medications are not a nursing action and one may hesitate to designate them as such on a form, but there is no denying that medications are a part of nursing action and need to be worked into a care plan somewhere. Medications can be an evolution, but often may also be an entropy when side effects and toxicity are considered.

A negative aspect relating to the sociocultural factors is identified as well. If the patient with a sociocultural difference is to function under a different culture's health care system, his differences must be considered an entropy. Intellectually, this can be accepted, but morally and ethically there are problems here. The same holds true with considering "postmenopause" an entropy, which is actually a sociocultural bias because of the emphasis placed on youth by this culture. These things are largely a matter of semantics and are not criticisms of the theory as such, but nurses should be more aware of subtle factors such as these.

One final criticism of the general systems theory plan is that it lacks a way to emphasize one area over another. It needs a way to designate the life-threatening situation factors as apart from those that are non–life-threatening (triage fashion).

Adaptations and Recommendations

This plan can avoid all the above-mentioned negative factors by simply remaining flexible. Freedom to add or delete categories as needed for individual patients should be emphasized. In addition, all areas need not be "maintained" should there exist no problem there; maintenance of some of these areas is beyond the scope of the nurse in a given situation. This would help nurses over the myth that they need to be all things to all people.

Repetition in the nursing plan can be avoided by referring to another area where the same problem is covered (e.g., "See under Circulation"). This demonstrates that the nurse has considered the fact that it may be a problem in several different systems but avoids redundancy.

Perhaps an interdisciplinary column would not be a bad idea. All multidisciplinary interventions could be noted together under the involved system, leaving the nursing action column clean for just pure nursing concerns (and we all know there are enough of these!). Items like consultations and medications could be noted in these additional columns.

A red star (or asterisk) system could be used to designate primary problem areas (like potentially life-threatening situations). Perhaps even placing the categories in the order of potential crisis to that patient would be helpful.

Conclusion

In summary, the general systems theory has good potential for use by the nursing profession, as it considers the patient as a whole in a multifaceted environment. The key to ironing out the few problems in the general systems theory is in keeping the whole plan functioning flexibly as this theory approaches individual patients.

III. A Critique of General Systems Theory

Deborah L. Oakes

General systems theory is a tool for assessing, planning, and evaluating patient problems, needs, and concerns. It is an excellent and valuable theory for use in the problem-solving process.

An imaginary scale of pros and cons has been devised as a critique. The weight readily tipped to the right, indicating the overwhelming advantages this theory has as opposed to its disadvantages. An attempt will be made here to relate both personal convictions about the theory and its applicability to the practice of nursing.

Man is a whole being, composed of many interrelating parts, each being dependent upon another for proper functioning and viability. The general systems theory attempts to look at the individual in his totality, scrutinizing all the components that go into the making of the "whole" being. The "wholeness" is kept intact while each unique yet interdependent aspect of man is analyzed.

Man exists in an open environment. Many forces are at work internally, as well as from the outside, to maintain him in a state of equilibrium. Negative forces are constantly striving to overcome the strengths of the system. Yet, in a healthy state, harmony between the two remains. Family situations, physical and environmental conditions, emotional stresses, bacterial invasions, etc., are just a small sample of the forces that can tip the balance into disequilibrium, or "dis-ease." When the negative forces (entropy) overcome man's positive assets or powers, evolution (a state of disharmony or illness) results.

This conceptual framework provides an essential guideline for all health-care providers. The general systems theory can be applied in any health/illness setting to assess the total patient/client. Delineating the components comprising the general system of man makes possible the ability to analyze the balance of forces, i.e., entropy versus evolution. Problems or disequilibrium can quickly be identified, goals established, and plans developed to return the scale to its balanced position.

Nurses as well as many other health team members frequently tend to view the patient as related to his physiological disease entity. The negative forces working on each component are easily identified and medical plans are devised and implemented to treat this one component or two; however, since man is a whole being, the many interrelating factors must also be considered. The disease processes could be affecting many unrecognized, not so apparent aspects. In like manner, many unnoticed factors could be affecting this disequilibrium state.

The general systems theory attempts to recognize all the influencing factors of man's open system. The all-too-frequently forgotten assets, strengths, and coping mechanisms can be supported and enhanced by the health team. Unrecognized problems can be more readily identified and necessary evolution resources implemented and encouraged.

The family plays an essential role in a patient's state of harmony (health). When the patient enters a state of disequilibrium, or illness, the entire family is affected; their own state of harmony is disturbed. The general systems theory considers the family's needs and also whether they can be supporting resources to the patient, or whether they are contributing to the patient's entropy.

The general systems theory is an excellent framework for assessing the entire patient unit (patient unit consisting of the patient, all significant others, and the environment). With even limited experience with the model, a vast amount of information can be collected about the patient unit that is pertinent to analyzing the negative forces as they oppose the existing positive assets. By delineating and weighing these two conflicting forces, areas that need assistance or support can be easily identified. Patient-centered goals are readily established and the actions needed to accomplish these goals clearly and briefly designated. The initial steps of the nursing process are incorporated into this theoretical tool.

But this conceptual model is not limited to the initial assessment of the patient. It can be an ongoing process of continual reevaluation and reassessment of problems, resources, outcomes, and revised plans of care. The general systems theory is unlimited in its use, being applicable throughout a patient's hospitalization, and following him into the community setting. It is an excellent means of assessing the patient's stage of learning and areas needed for discharge planning and patient education.

The general systems theory amplifies the nurses' professional judgment, problem-solving, and decision-making processes. Professional knowledge must be employed, utilizing scientific rationale for understanding the underlying pathological processes, the influencing factors, and the actions which are needed to rectify the problems and to support the evolutionary assets. Being a *systematic* appraisal of the whole patient unit – bio-psycho-social – the complete nursing process is enhanced and ensured.

Another plus for this theoretical model is its ability to establish priorities readily. With the underlying imbalances clearly stated, a hierarchy of needed actions can be identified.

Though other members of the health team were not enlisted in the author's personal use of this tool in assessing various patients, this is an all-important possibility. The general systems theory is easily understood and, once explained, not only the theoretical framework but also the tool could be used by all health team personnel. Continuity of care will be facilitated and ensured. All health/illness settings, and all disciplines of health professionals can find this theory a major step forward in their patient care.

The general systems theory is easy to complete, requiring very little time, at least in comparison to previously used tools. Short, simple phrases can be employed, making it more appealing not only to those who must complete the form but also to those personnel who are "too busy" to read lengthy reports. It can be a reference source, being so delineated that needed data may be obtained at a quick glance. All health team members may be more willing to utilize this tool considering the two important factors of brevity and time conservation.

This theoretical framework is flexible and practical in all health settings. The outpatient medicine clinic, a medical unit, and even home care proved to be excellent areas for employing this tool. Excitement grew about a tool which, for once, was completely understood and found exceptionally applicable, and the decision was made to try it on patients other than mainly medical-surgical. In doing a mini-research study in the labor and delivery unit, a few of the patient's points of entropy versus evolution were quickly recorded. The woman chosen for this was a young primigravida, preeclamptic patient. Limited experience with postpartum mothers was a disadvantage, but the author found this tool easy to employ and quite useful. This mini-experiment confirmed the belief that all health disciplines will find this tool to be a major asset in improving the quality of patient care.

Additional categories can easily be inserted into this model where needed. Personal hygiene was a very important aspect of care for the diabetic patient who was followed. This could be included in the body integrity category. However, since hygiene is such an important aspect of care, a separate section is more appropriate.

At times, some categories were redundant but this can be justified since the patient is a "whole" being and all components are interrelated. The nursing actions tended to overlap or be repeated in several sections, but that was mainly evident in the Nursing Concerns area. Safety and Instruction were previously incorporated in the preceding individual categories under Physiological and Psychosocial Needs. The Nursing Concerns category was confusing to me on the whole. The semantics of what is a nursing concern was not clearly understood. Is the concern of the nurse safety, instruction, and coordination of care? Or are these additional actions or functions that one must strive to fulfill? Safety and Instruction can be included in the prior categories, Coordination of care being listed under *patient* needs as a separate entity. If special problems with safety or instruction – e.g., high anxiety, extreme pain, etc. – were found, additional categories could then be inserted.

One aspect of the Newman model which was found to be extremely worthwhile was the patient's input and perceptions of his illness, needs, and goals. Though this can and should be a part of the general systems theory, special instructions and sample questions may be a guide to nurses for completing this all-too-frequently forgotten area. The author strongly believes that most assessments and plans of care should be done *with* the patient and family. Their expectations, perceptions and preferences *must* be considered. The general systems theory does allow for this but constant reminders are needed by many people. Clear-cut guidelines for patient input would be a valuable asset to this theoretical tool.

In summary, the author has found both the theory and tool applicable, efficient, comprehensive, and very practical. The utilization of general systems theory creates an enrichment of thought processes. Colleagues are encouraged and challenged to embark on this rewarding experience. With continued use, suggestions for improvements, and minor revisions, the general systems theory will prove to be a step toward the ultimate goal of improvement of the quality of nursing care.

Applicability of General Systems Theory to the Nursing System

13

I. General Systems Theory and Nursing Service

Arlene M. Putt

Use By Staff Nurses

Mesarovic [2] listed the following five functions of general systems theory:

1. Unify various branches of systems theory
2. Aid in applying the systems models to new areas
3. Provide a precise language for multidisciplinary problems and interdisciplinary communications
4. Provide a means for describing large-scale systems
5. Permit synthesis and organization of human knowledge in rather diverse but still related areas

The general systems theory statement should be mathematically precise – but not restrictive – and simply formulated.

With the above points as a guide, how practical are the general systems concepts for nursing by general-duty nurses who have no background in the theoretical framework?

To test this applicability, general-duty nurses were selected from among those working on a 43-bed general medical unit of a large metropolitan hospital. With the head nurse's knowledge and support, one nurse at a time was selected to try out the assessment format. The author spent about 45 minutes explaining the basic concepts and how to use the assessment guide. Then the nurse who indicated her willingness to give the format a try would, in the course of her duties, assess a variety of patients using the assessment guide. At a later time, the author returned to review with the nurse her experiences in trying to utilize the format. In the meantime, the assessments made were available to other members of the nursing team for their use. One unplanned incident indicated how the assessment could be utilized. An oncoming evening nurse was called to the phone to give a report on a patient who was being transferred. The nurse had not had time to familiarize herself with the patient's condition. Available to her was the assessment on that particular patient. With this in hand, the evening nurse gave a concise but complete report as judged by the head nurse, who witnessed the incident. The evening nurse's comment after the incident was that the assessment guide was very helpful.

The value of any assessment tool is related to its currency. As with any other nursing care plan, the information must be revalidated and readjusted as frequently as the patient's state of functioning or his circumstances change. With a form that can be done in pencil and can be redone in a few minutes, the pressure of time need not be a deterrent to use. The old pragmatic chance identification of patient problems and nursing approaches is not adequate for planning quality nursing care. Through the use of this assessment guide, the patient data are systematically processed through an understanding of the forces at work, thus providing sound rationale for professional nursing care. In this way, nursing practice and nursing theory validate each other.

Applicability to Peer Review

With the advent of peer review committees, the need for a systematic approach to ascertain the completeness of care becomes a necessity. The general systems theory nursing care plan lends itself to this use with the minor adaptation of a column in which to record expected outcome of the nursing action. To date this use of the general systems theory nursing care plan has not been tested practice, but the thought is worthy of consideration.

Along the same line of thinking, the general systems theory nursing care plan could be used to develop standardized care plans which could be available with minor adaptation to the patient upon admission to the unit or clinic. A standardized plan would give the nurse an additional reference against which to determine if all the patient's needs have been assessed and care has been initiated.

Applicability to Problem-oriented Medical Records

The general systems process described is readily adaptable for use with problem-oriented recording. In problem-oriented medical records, the patient's problems are identified and listed numerically. Each time a note is added, the problem is addressed by number and name and the information is organized according to subjective and objective data categories with an assessment as to the state of the problem and a plan of action, These parts of the problem discussion are abbreviated S, O, A , and P. This method of record development, originated by Weed [4], and described by Bjorn and Cross [1] and Schell and Campbell [3], is widely utilized in medical centers.

Problem-oriented Medical Record

Problem
Number
Name
Type
  Physiological
  Psychosocial
  Nursing

Data
Subjective
  Entropy
  Evolution
Objective
  Entropy
  Evolution

Assessment
State of problem
Goal

Plan
Medical approach
Nursing intervention

Evaluation
Reassessment

Figure 6. Application of general systems concepts to problem-oriented records

The general systems concepts could be included in this method of recording. The patient problem might be identified as to type of problem such as physiological, psychosocial, or nursing concern. Descriptions of the entropy and evolution present in the problem could be included with the subjective and objective data categories. The assessment section presents an evaluation of the balance of the forces. The plan of action synthesizes the goal (equifinality) with the actions outlined to achieve that goal. Periodic updating of the problem necessitates reassessment and evaluation of the situation with adjustment as indicated.

An attempt to combine these concepts into a usable tool is illustrated in Figure 6. Credit is given to Lynn Hicks for partial development of this integration. To clarify the concepts more fully, a case study in problem-oriented style follows.

References

1. Bjorn, J. C., and Cross, H. D. *The Problem-oriented Private Practice of Medicine.* Chicago: Modern Hospital Press, 1970.
2. Mesarovic, M. A Mathematical Theory of General Systems. In G. Klir (Ed.), *Trends in General Systems Theory.* New York: John Wiley and Sons, 1972.

3. Schell, P., and Campbell, A. T. POMR: Not just another way to chart. *Nurs. Outlook* 20:510, 1972.
4. Weed, L. L. *Medical Records, Medical Education and Patient Care.* Cleveland: Case University Press, 1969.

II. A Family Affair — with Dignity and Serenity

Lois E. Prosser

The family is a critical human system distinguished by its goals, functions, and climate of feeling. It is a social system of individuals with whom each person interacts and performs family functions. There are situations when a family requires assistance from health-care professionals to adapt to personal and environmental stresses. Assessing the dynamic relationships between the family and the health care providers is a social systems approach of interacting elements. Community health nursing practice is family-oriented; it provides the perspective of intervention possibilities, either to work toward helping the family adjust to its social situations or attempt to change the social situation so that it will be less stressful to the individual family members.

This section will describe meaningful concepts of social interaction theory based on community health nursing practice. A case study using the problem-oriented approach illustrates a way of thinking about, describing, and evaluating the effectiveness of nursing intervention for a family coping with death.

Buckley defined a system as "a complex of elements or components directly or indirectly related in a causal network, such that each component is related to at least some others in a more or less stable way within a particular period of time" [2, p. 41]. A general systems approach is a way of looking at and thinking about selected aspects of family and clinical nursing interaction. The clinical aspects of family/nurse behavior could be described as a *holon.* This term is borrowed from Koestler [4], who used it to express the idea that each social entity is simultaneously a part and a whole. Koestler suggested that a holon faces two directions at once – inward toward its own parts, and outward to the system of which it is a part [4]. If a family and the community health nurse are viewed as a holon, attention must be given to all the persons involved within the social situation, assessing the changes and the effects that occur in the environment, recognizing that events are relative to the position of the observer. What occurs in social systems are "transfers of energy" between persons. The energy in this dynamic process may not be directly observable but inferred from the effects of the system and its parts. Anderson and Carter [1] defined energy as "capacity for action," "action," or "power to effect change." They also suggest that information and resources are potential energy. Energy is the prime function of a social system. Energy and information are complementary. Energy draws from a complex of sources; physical capacity of members; social resources such as loyalties, shared sentiments and common values, ideas, and manpower.

The process of multiplication of energy is *synergy*. This process is appropriate to describing an open system through absorption of new stimuli and constant adaptation to the environment with stimulus of new ideas and attachments. The behavioral aspects of a social system indicate social control through bargaining. The introduction of a nurse to a distressed family provides the energy to explore alternatives to cope with stressful situations; she acts as a catalyst to the decision-making objective.

Family care is more complex by nature than individual care because of the many interacting personalities, the needs of the group, and the need for decisions about problems that affect everyone in a different way. In addition, there are situational variables, environmental influences, needs and desires, perceptual conflicts and expectations of the health care system as well as the health care providers. The introduction of nursing in the management of families suggests an intermediary between elements of several social systems interacting simultaneously. Nursing is the energy factor in collecting and interpreting data toward defining the problem, suggesting alternative solutions, accepting the decisions of the family based on personal preference, implementing the decisions, and evaluating the effectiveness of the strategies. The dynamics of community health nursing are directed toward adaptive changes in the family, the nurse's interaction and the health care situation. The nurse's roles are multifaceted. The roles can be discrete or blend with each other to accomplish the goals of maintenance of family integrity. The roles can be those of facilitator, advocate, consultant, teacher, counselor, therapeutic interventionist and/or primary care provider. The nurse's roles are to assist in overcoming hurdles, to initiate potential capacity to function in an acceptable way, and to react to the present so as to plan realistically for the future. This implies recognition of the potential of individuals within the family group, their strengths, and their weaknesses.

The nurse influences the actions of the family that is seeking health care. She controls environmental factors by removing restrictions, providing information for decision-making, and by helping to perform actions to achieve goals. Nursing, as defined by King [3, p. 89], is critical to community health nursing practice. "Nursing is a process of action, reaction, interaction, and transaction whereby nurses assist individuals of any age and socioeconomic group to meet their basic needs in performing activities of daily living and to cope with health and illness at some particular point in the life cycle." Inferences are made from thoughts and feelings, words and acts. The perceptions, judgments, actions, and reactions of both nurse and family determine the transactions of the situations. Transactions occur when a reciprocal relationship is established between the nurse and the family in which both actively participate in determining goals to be achieved in specific situations. The transactional process is the essence of nursing practice as described in the American Nurses' Association Standards of Community Health Nursing. Participation of the individual and family in goal determination is required.

During the interactive process of nursing care, human behavior can be analyzed through perceptual determinants of sociocultural factors, psychological factors, and physiological factors. Communication of observed phenomena is utilized to facilitate interaction among the individuals and systems involved in the influence of change toward adaptation toward a steady state.

A family study illustrates a social systems approach to community health nursing process. The situation is one that faces every family sometime – the death of a family member.

In the Middle Ages, a dying man was the central focus of control of his life. Preparation for death was based on the reality of a "good death." In this instance, the dying man performed many functions; he blessed his children; forgave his enemies; repented his sins in a personal manner; and planned his funeral in great detail. Today, this part of living is unusual. It is unusual because of the techniques and knowledge of medical intervention, the use of the hospital for critical care of patients paid for by medical insurance, and limited experience of families to make decisions in such a crisis. For those selected families who are given the opportunity to make decisions about care in the final stages of illness, the community health nurse, by her preparation and experience, is able to manipulate the situation, the systems involved, and the environment. She creates the atmosphere and the setting for the dying person and his family to face death with dignity, care, comfort and serenity. Seeking the "good death" and support in *ars mortende* (art of dying) for both the family and the client is a challenge. The author had the opportunity to know such a family and a situation. She became "involved" in various roles with a family who recognized the problem and who sought assistance to reach their goals. The information will be presented through the problem-oriented format with adaptations for family care. The problems are identified as family-oriented rather than person-oriented – general rather than specific. Emphasis is placed on the nursing process of perception, judgment, action, and reaction, leading to transaction of problem-solving.

A family profile is presented, as well as a brief description of the situation at each nursing encounter. The problem-oriented approach is the mechanism utilized to present explanatory data. Objective evidence is presented first inasmuch as inferences are made by the nurse on situational data rather than medical data. These inferences are based on perceptions and judgments. The subjective data confirm or change the judgments and verify the assessments. Plans are the actions, reactions, and transactions of the problem-solving process. The focus will be on family human needs and the nursing process rather than on medical needs. A final paragraph describes the beginning resolution of the grieving process. Both the family and the nurse grew in their personal capacities and level of competence during the intense period of caring for and comforting Mr. J. in accomplishing his death with dignity and serenity.

Family Profile

Mr. J., a 53-year-old professor of business and public administration, had lived for the past 15 years in one community: the year of his illness, he was on sabbatical leave. Much of his personal and professional life had been devoted to numerous community endeavors. He was intellectually curious and displayed concern for his fellow man.

Mrs. J., a 52-year-old housewife, was graduated from a business college over 20 years ago. She is confined to a wheelchair as a result of poliomyelitis in 1955, with residual paralysis of both legs, but is able to perform all her household functions well. She has maintained her integrity and vitality through the love and devotion of her husband and two sons and a strong support system of many friends. During this time she has maintained a strong outside interest in and commitment to the arts in the community.

The older son, a 21-year-old senior university student in a neighboring state, was described by his mother as sensitive, conscientious, and studious. The younger son, a 19-year-old sophomore university student in his home town, volunteers many hours helping youth with sports activities. He has many friends and significant others in his life; one of them is the coach of the basketball team. There are two pets in the family – Jiggs, a 12-year-old brown-black and white bulldog, is a constant companion to Mrs. J., and Cho, a 10-year-old multicolored long-haired cat, is independent and curious.

The home of the J. family is located in a residential neighborhood about a 10-minute drive from the hospital. The house has three bedrooms, a large kitchen, two bathrooms, a laundry area, and a large living room. The house was designed by Mr. J. to accommodate life with a wheelchair. The yard is enclosed by a concrete block wall that provides privacy for users of the swimming pool in the back of the house. The view from the kitchen and living room is a spectacular one of a nearby mountain range.

Resources. The family is financially sound with an unusually fine hospitalization policy provided by the University; this plan covered all contingencies. There is a strong support system of friends and colleagues who are in constant touch with all family members. The church is a vital part of the lives of this family.

Situation. Mr. J. had been receiving medical care for a variety of physical problems during the past 5 years. Until the past year he was quite healthy. During this interval of time, Mr. J. was able to teach full time and actively participated in his numerous outside activities. He exercised, maintained a good diet, did not smoke, and his weight was average for his height and build. During the past year, he had been hospitalized 5 times for diagnosis and treatment of cancer of the lung with metastasis to the bone and brain. He had adapted to radiation therapy, chemotherapy, and physical therapy during the course of his illness. At the time of nursing intervention, a crisis had developed when the physician announced on Saturday that Mr. J. was to be discharged on Monday. The family was not consulted about the discharge plans. A friend of the family called Sunday morning asking for help.

Problem. Loss of intactness of family faced with death; feeling of hopelessness.

Home Visit

On December 15 the author made a home visit.

Objective Data. Mrs. J. opened the door. Her face was tearstained and her eyes brimming; her hands were shaking, she seemed somewhat breathless, and her appearance was disheveled. She wheeled her chair in a backward and forward motion in a purposeless fashion. The dog remained at her side during the 2½-hour interview.

Subjective Data. Mrs. J. stated that she was not prepared to have her husband discharged from the hospital on Monday; she had been unable to tell the physician about her doubts; there were too many plans to be made; and at this time she was unable to "think straight." Information was shared that both Mr. and Mrs. J. knew the diagnosis, as well as the boys; however, they did not know the expected time of death. She had been told Mr. J. might live for from 6 months to a year. When confronted with asking for a personal judgment, since she had been living with him for 30 years and knew him better than anyone, she sighed deeply and said, "I estimate about six weeks; he is very weak and I don't know if I can manage alone. We have discussed the possibility of my husband's dying at home – I want to take care of him; he was so good to me during my long illness with polio, but I don't know if I can."

Assessment. Explore alternatives to care: (1) home care, (2) nursing home care, (3) Veterans' Hospital care. Eligibility and financial constraints were clarified.

Plans

1. Arrange for home care because Mr. J. refused to go to a nursing home
2. Make a list of equipment and supplies needed for care at home
3. Act as advocate in hospital system to delay discharge a few days to implement plan 2
4. Clarify wishes of Mr. J. in the decision-making process
5. Plan for part-time nursing care through the Visiting Nurse Association until full-time care is needed

Problem. Clarify options available for the family with the hospital system and with Mr. J.

The Next Day

Objective Data – Hospital System. Discharge plan for December 16 recorded on chart.

Subjective Data. Consulted with physicians about inopportune time for discharge; related knowledge of information from visit to home on Sunday emphasizing the need for adequate planning. Learned that although a 6-month period had been presented to Mrs. J., 6 weeks would be a more realistic estimate.

Shared with the medical personnel that this was Mrs. J.'s estimate as well – their reaction one of surprise. Negotiated postponement of discharge until Mr. J. could be included in the decision-making. Agreement secured with reluctance. Asked for prescriptions for needs (1–4).

1. Electric hospital bed with special gel-foam mattress
2. Medications
3. Special mouth care needs
4. Commode
5. Clarify source of medical care at home when needed
6. Make referral to Visiting Nurse Association

Objective Data – Mr. J. Patient lying in hospital bed with no acute distress, but was very pale, lips cracked, appeared weak with untouched breakfast tray at bedside. Eyes were closed, breathing normal.

Subjective Data. Introduced self and talked about conversation with his wife yesterday about discharge plans.

Presented alternatives. Mr. J. became upset with both prospects – nursing home or Veterans' Hospital care. His preference was home care. Then he asked, "Can you tell me how long it will be?" Response was, "Not really, but I can give you a professional judgment – 6 weeks or longer; however, you must remember that when you go home, your family and I will provide all the comfort you need, not cure." We held hands and cried together for some minutes. When asked when he wanted to go home he replied, "Wednesday, about 3:00 PM. By then the sun will be shining and the wind will have died down."

Assessment. Discharge hospital plans completed with input from all systems concerned. Explore alternatives for transportation:

1. Ambulance
2. Automobile
3. Special van

Plans

1. Secure prescriptions for equipment and medications
2. Write referral for Visiting Nurse Association obtaining physician's signature
3. Interpret decision of family for discharge on Wednesday afternoon at 3:00 PM to physicians and nursing staff in spite of usual procedure of early morning discharges
4. Phone Mrs. J. about Mr. J.'s decision; give her list of equipment needed and where she could find them
5. Assist in mobilizing resources if Mrs. J. is unable to handle herself
6. Plan for part-time nursing care consistent with needs of client and family

7. Explore preference of mode of transportation (judgment of nurse and physician is ambulance)

Second Hospital Visit

Objective Data. Mr. J. was sitting up in bed and seemed relaxed although weak. Physical condition unchanged.

Subjective Data. When given the alternative choices of transportation, Mr. J. was emphatic about not going home in an ambulance; strong personal integrity evident. He elected to have a friend, who usually drove his wife, take him home in Mrs. J.'s wheelchair. The friend had a van designed for that specific purpose complete with ramp. We discussed where he wished to have his hospital bed at home. He replied, "In the living room, of course. There I will have a beautiful view of the mountains and a fireplace that is special to me." At this point, his wife came in and said in a clear voice, "Dear, I am going to fix up my bedroom for you, won't that be nice?" He sighed and turned his head in disappointment. It appeared that decisions were being made for him without consideration of his personal preference. I presented the plans Mr. J. and I had discussed. The living room was his preference. I suggested that we could try this on an experimental basis and move him if it did not work out. I explained the meaningfulness of being in the middle of family involvement. There were a few minutes of silence; then she asked her husband if that was what he really wanted. He said, "Please."

Assessment. Needs of the client were explicit for method of transportation; home and room preference clarified.

Plans

1. Have Mrs. J. call her friend to bring Mr. J. home on Wednesday
2. Visit home to make bed and arrange equipment for home care
3. Include boys in planning for lifting father into his bed when we get home
4. Arrange time to accompany Mr. J. in van for trip home since his wife would be unable to do this
5. Interpret choice of transportation to physician and plans for safety

Problem. Safe, secure action for transfer from hospital to home environment.

The Return Home

Objective Data. On December 18, the personal friend of Mrs. J. and I met in the hospital room at 3:00 PM. We transferred Mr. J. to Mrs. J.'s wheelchair, collected personal belongings, and said brief good-byes to the staff. It took 10 minutes to get through the hospital and into the van. Mr. J. remained straight in his chair, with no discernible changes in vital signs. The trip home took an additional 10 minutes in bright sunshine and very little traffic. Mr. J. expressed his thanks to his wife's friend for her willingness to provide the needed transportation, expressing again his displeasure with the thought of an ambulance ride. Upon arrival at home, Mrs. J., both boys, and the animals were waiting outside. As the wheelchair came off the ramp, the cat jumped into Mr. J.'s lap, the dog barked joyously, Mrs. J. smiled with tears in her eyes, and the boys watched the interactions with smiles on their faces. The younger son wheeled his father's chair into the living room. As planned, the boys picked up their father and placed him in his hospital bed. This was their first attempt, so he landed on his face and abdomen in bed. Everybody laughed and tension was released. With the help of the boys we changed his position and made him comfortable. An electric buzzer had been installed by a friend of the younger son's with adhesive tape to the bedside stand.

Problem. Comfort and special care needs.

Subjective Data. Mrs. J. asked how to manage her husband's medication regimen. A notebook was found to record times of medication and explanations for use of each item were given. An index page was developed describing the medications; a separate page was designated for each day with time to be recorded.

Multiple vitamins – 1 daily
Nitrofurantoin (Macrodantin) for mouth care – p.r.n.
Acetaminophen (Tylenol) – tabs 2 q3 or 4h p.r.n.
Hydromorphone (Dilaudid) – tab 1 q4h p.r.n.
Flurazepam (Dalmane) – 1 capsule at bedtime, to be repeated × 1 p.r.n.
Fleet's enema – p.r.n.

Mr. J. suggested that Tylenol was preferable to him. Mr. J., Mrs. J., and I discussed the use and action of acetaminophen and hydromorphone to control discomfort and pain. Mr. J. reasserted his preference for acetaminophen. It seemed to provide the comfort needed at the time. When acetaminophen was no longer useful, he would ask for hydromorphone by mouth. He agreed to the plan.

Plans

1. General care tomorrow
2. Demonstrate back care and special mouth care
3. Discuss good preferences and value of small feedings

Home Visit

Objective Data. On December 19, Mr. J. was in bed raised at 90-degree angle reading student papers. Color good, vital signs normal. T., 98.2°F; P., 62 regular; R., 18, BP 120/80. Abdomen soft, weight 130. Gums, lips, and teeth coated with dried blood.

Subjective Data. Mr. J. stated he had the best night of rest in five weeks without sleeping pills, had not needed to use the buzzer, had enjoyed his breakfast and was planning to sit in his favorite chair today. He had taken Tylenol twice since my visit yesterday.

Special Care. Bed bath given. Skin clear except for mild redness over sacral protuberances. Demonstrated back care with lotion to the two sons, and need to keep sheets free of wrinkles. They agreed to do this 3 times a day or more often if Dad asked for it. Demonstrated mouth care with use of a toothette, removing old blood and applying vaseline to lips. Mr. J. then stood up, his balance was excellent, and he took a few steps to his favorite chair. Bed was changed.

Discussed nutrition needs with both Mr. and Mrs. J. He was not hungry, but agreed to try six small meals a day. Explored preferences of soft foods because of sensitivity of mouth and gums.

Plans

1. Visit three times weekly for assessment, general care, mouth care, and enemas p.r.n.
2. Family to call if help was needed on an interim basis

This arrangement worked well for 2 weeks. Mouth ulcerations healing with special mouth care and regular ingestion of yogurt. Mr. J. was up twice every day but for shorter periods of time. Persistent pain in his back necessitated Dilaudid. The family provided excellent nursing care for Mr. J. At the end of 2 weeks when Mr. J. was not strong enough to get out of bed and unable to swallow medications by mouth another family problem occurred.

Problem. Secure injectable hydromorphone.

Later Stages

Objective Data. On January 2, the physician refused to provide needles and syringes for pain medication; requested rehospitalization if Mr. J. was this incapacitated.

Subjective Data. Discussed decision of physician with family and inability of nurse to convince the physician that Mr. J. really wanted to remain at home. Mrs. J. was upset and asked what hospitalization would mean. Told her he would receive his pain medication by hypodermic route, possibly oxygen as required, full nursing care and possibly life-saving measures. She cried and asked, "What for – what will it mean?" Suggested a few additional weeks of life and less stress for her and the boys. She said "No, we have done so well and he really wants to die at home. What can I do?" Suggested she call the physician and tell him her decision since I obviously was unable to change the system. That afternoon, syringes, needles and injectable hydromorphone were delivered to me.

Plans

1. Reevaluate needs of patient and family
2. Teach administration of medication
3. Continue care on a daily basis until plans for private-duty nursing could be implemented

Problem. Full-time nursing care needed.

Objective Data. On January 4, Mr. J. was now confined to bed 24 hours a day. He required hydromorphone 4 to 6 times daily. He was unable to move easily. Vital signs: T., 97.2°F; P., 100; R., 28; BP, 90/60. Mouth clear and clean but dry as a result of mouth-breathing.

Subjective Data. Mrs. J. and the boys finally revealed that they were unable to provide constant 24-hour care. They were all becoming tired and short-tempered as a result of continuing vigilance. They also admitted not being prepared for death without support although Kübler-Ross' book *On Death and Dying* had been most helpful.

Assessment. Full-time nursing care needed because of family wishes and condition of Mr. J.

Plans

1. Discontinue part-time nursing care
2. Develop nursing care plan for private-duty nurses
3. Arrange for availability of nursing consultation for private-duty nurses by telephone or home visits
4. Be available to family members p.r.n.
5. Secure written orders from physician for full-time nursing services consistent with requirements of health care policy
6. Plan for funeral arrangements

Problem. Death with dignity and serenity.

On January 19, private-duty nurses with experience caring for cancer patients were secured to begin immediately on a 24-hour basis. The family felt great relief but continued to spend periods of time talking with Mr. J. as we had planned. They also took turns feeding him and giving small amounts of fluid. Mrs. J. frequently held his hand even when he was unable to respond to her. The last day of Mr. J.'s life, Mrs. J. called to have me evaluate the competence of a substitute nurse who had arrived because of illness of the regular private-duty nurse. Reassurance was given after observation. When Mrs. J. was reassured, we again discussed funeral arrangements. Mrs. J. stated that she had contacted the funeral director, who would stop at the hospital to have the final evaluation made there; the cost was $250. This she was willing to do. The pattern of living had slowed down to a gentle quiet. Mr. J. died on February 18 in peace. Mrs. J. said, "We really did it, didn't we? This is just what my husband wanted. I am so pleased that our plans were able to be fulfilled."

On February 20, received a special call from Mrs. J. to attend the memorial services and come to the house following services. The church was full of friends and associates. The service was warm and meaningful. Six men discussed Mr. J.'s contribution to the community and the University. Over a hundred people came to the house to help Mrs. J. and her sons accept this recent loss of husband and father. Mrs. J. introduced me to the majority of their friends explaining how she had been able to provide her husband with his preference in dying at home because of my help. The boys spent an hour talking with me about the meaning of their father's death as well as their plans for the future. They had not realized how comforting it would be to assist with their father's care and how much the community recognized him for his contributions. They had not looked at him as a special person, rather as the authority figure who punished them when they misbehaved as children or insisted that they maintain good grades in school.

All family members had adapted to this crisis in their lives and were comforted through their participation in activities and decisions that affected them all. As the nurse providing both energy and synergy in a complex social situation, I, too, believed and demonstrated that nursing makes a difference. Many roles were initiated throughout the intense involvement with a family of many strengths, yet they could not cope well with the diversity of the goals of a health care system. This case presentation reveals the need for a facilitator, an advocate, and consultant as well as a therapeutic interventionist, primary care provider, teacher, and counselor. The blend of the roles culminated in transactions to help the family meet their needs. The interactions of this family system, the nursing systems, and the medical systems suggest that any one system is not sufficient to change the environment and the situation for healthy resolutions. The behavior of everyone is contingent upon interpretations of events. Certainly the interaction of the family and the community health nurse developed into a holon – with the nurse becoming a part of the family during the events of a death with dignity and serenity.

References

1. Anderson, R., and Carter, I. *Human Behavior in the Social Environment: A Social Systems Approach.* Chicago: Aldine Publishing, 1974.
2. Buckley, W. (Ed.). *Modern Systems Research for the Behavioral Scientist.* Chicago: Aldine Publishing, 1968.
3. King, I. *Toward a Theory for Nursing: General Concepts of Human Behavior.* New York: John Wiley & Sons, 1971.
4. Koestler, A., and Smythes, J. R. *Beyond Reductionism: New Perspectives in the Life Sciences.* Boston: Beacon Press, 1971.

III. General Systems Theory and Nursing Research

Arlene M. Putt

Systematic research into patient care can be guided by an understanding of the universal processes described in general systems theory, identifying and quantifying the processes, and then manipulating the expansion, contraction, or stabilization of the processes with quantification of the results. Here is where experimental design may be applied. Identification and quantification of the processes can be achieved through systematic assessment of the system in which the processes are operating, which, in the case of patient care, is the patient, his family, and community. Whatever the system, it can be divided into logical subsystems for purposes of analysis. The continuums of entropy and evolution can be divided into subunits, and each subsystem can be measured or evaluated on each continuum with the obtained data being either parametric or nonparametric, depending upon the nature of the system. For instance, a patient's biopsychosocial functioning may be conceived as a set of physiological systems, a set of psychological systems, and a set of social or cultural systems which are operating in concert at a given time in a given situation. The patient's physiological systems may be divided into as minute a unit as desired for study and analysis. One subsystem may be explored and manipulated while holding other systems constant to the degree that they can be stabilized when they are part of an interacting chain.

If one wishes to study the patient's respiratory functioning as a system, the patient's functioning may be analyzed in terms of partial pressures of gases, amount of oxygen consumed, or other measures such as the volumes of gases exchanged. His state of entropy and his evolutionary potential in relation to respiratory function can be quantified, the experimental variables applied and the function reevaluated.

Because single factors seldom operate in isolation, multiple classification techniques of analysis of variance or multiple regression procedures might be very useful in assisting with the interpretations of interacting factors. The key is to approach the problems in a thorough, systematic fashion. To date, much research in nursing has been sporadic in nature. The tendency has been to develop studies of one aspect of patient care without regard as to how this aspect fits into the total picture of man interacting with his total environment. The proposal to examine systematically successive aspects of care is an arduous one but essential if studies are to have meaningful relationships to each other. The computer should be utilized to work out the possible permutations for study; these could then be explored in succession. Collaborative studies could hasten the process as long as comparable frameworks and measurements were utilized. This scheme for designing future nursing research is on a grand scale, but grossly complex problems such as befall health care at the present time require bigger and better conceived solutions. Utilization of a general systems framework for nursing research could put reason and organization into the search for truth where little exists at the present time.

Glossary of Terms Used in General Systems Theory

agency: a term used by Dickoff, James, and Weidenbach to mean the performer of the action
assessment: the gathering of data and the interpretation of the data in relation to the present situation of the patient
closed system: a functioning unit isolated from its surrounding environment with no interaction with the environment
concept: an idea of something formed by combining its characteristics
construct: complex concepts
dynamics: a term used by Dickoff, James, and Weidenbach to mean the type and amount of energies utilized
entropy: the tendency to increased randomness by the dissipation of energy; the running down of a system
equifinality: the sameness of the end result starting from various points; the sameness of the goal
evolution: the process of developing higher organization and complexity; the counterforce to entropy
feedback: the return of a small amount of the output of a system to the input so as to correct and guide further output
framework: a term used by Dickoff, James, and Weidenbach to mean the context of the situation
general systems: a collection of general concepts, principles, problems, and techniques associated with systems
general systems theory: the scientific exploration of wholes and wholeness
gestalt: a complete, whole, unanalyzable pattern of experience, perceived as such
hierarchy: a system of ranking one thing above another in order of power or control
holon: a social entity simultaneously a part and a whole
integration: merging of parts into a whole or total organism
isomorphism: parallelism that occurs in totally different systems
multifinality: multiple outcomes dependent upon the selected means

negative entropy: the counterforce to entropy, also referred to in the literature as negentropy; synonymous with evolution as utilized by this author
open system: a unit of functioning that interacts freely with its environment
patiency: a term used by Dickoff, James, and Weidenbach to mean the recipient of the action
principle: two or more concepts linked together in a statement of relationship
problem-oriented record: a method of organizing medical records to facilitate the recording and finding of information and the identification and handling of medical problems as originated by Weed
servo-dynamic mechanism: a subsystem of interrelated parts that serves to keep the system energetic
servo-mechanism: a mechanism that serves a purpose within the system
S.O.A.P.: abbreviations for subjective, objective, assessment, and plans, the parts of the workup of the problem within the problem-oriented medical record
synergy: the process of multiplication of energy
terminus: a term used by Dickoff, James, and Weidenbach to mean the end point of the activity

Index

DATE DU
Demco, Inc. 38-293
GAYLORD